FACTORS UNFORESEEN

About the Author

Harvey Shoals was born 27 January 1922 on a small farm south of Burlington, Vermont. After WWII, while attending college on the GI Bill, he majored in biology and then continued for a doctorate in field biology and epidemiology. ***Factors Unforeseen*** traces his role during 1958 and 1959 to find an environmentally safe way to control a deadly, parasitic, tropical disease on the island of Tavira in the Caribbean, a role that went hopelessly awry and nearly cost him his life.

FACTORS

UNFORESEEN

by

Harvey Shoals

Infinity Publishing
Haverford, PA

ISBN 0-7414-1649-2

Published by:

INFINITY
PUBLISHING.COM

519 West Lancaster Avenue
Haverford, PA 19041-1413
Info@buybooksontheweb.com
www.buybooksontheweb.com
Toll-free (877) BUY BOOK
Local Phone (610) 520-2500
Fax (610) 519-0261

Printed in the United States of America

Printed on Recycled Paper

Published July 2003

for

Maggie

The author wishes to thank Doreen Gandy Wiley and Pamela Masters for many helpful suggestions regarding the text, and William Rowan for designing the cover.

FLIGHT

TO AGUILAS

Nearly half a century has passed since my assignment to the island of Tavira in the Caribbean. I'm not especially proud of the part I played in what happened there. I should have distanced myself emotionally from the undercurrent of political confusion that surfaced soon after I arrived.

I was sent to Tavira by the Parasitic Diseases Section (PDS) of the World Health Organization to advise the government with a problem of disease control, but, progressively, in order to achieve certain of my goals, I allowed myself to take sides on a matter that had nothing to do with my assignment.

Without applying too much hindsight, one could say that I simply failed to understand the politics of change.

The year was 1958. As a young field biologist, thirty-six and single—debatably single—I had just completed a fantastically exciting two-year assignment in tropical Africa, and I had just begun a two-year hitch in Puerto Rico when George Barlow at the PDS headquarters in Geneva suddenly pulled me out of Puerto Rico and reassigned me to the island of Tavira to replace a biologist that the Tavirans had abruptly deported.

On the flight from San Juan, Puerto Rico to Aguilas, Tavira, I penned the following letter to Sam Tyler back at the Tropical Disease Field Research Station in San Juan. During the previous nine days, Sam and I had been working together near the sugar cane fields south and southeast of San Juan close to Guayama and Humacao where the Puerto Rican health department was experiencing a severe outbreak of a waterborne disease with the informal name of *snail fever*.

Sam knew that snail fever was most prevalent in the streamside villages where, with few exceptions, the owners of the sugar cane *centrales* (factories) allowed their workers to build homes. These dwellings barely qualified as homes. Tin roofed and raised on stilts, they were typical of the shanties of impoverished laborers not only of the Caribbean, but in tropical nations throughout the world. The women of these villages washed their clothes at streamside, pounding them on smooth stones to force soap through the weave of the cloth, while their infants and small children splashed at play, oblivious to the danger lurking in those warm pools of crystal clear water.

Sam had been studying snail fever in Puerto Rico for a couple of years. I'd been looking forward to working with him, and was sorely disappointed to be suddenly flown out to Tavira.

In 1950, Sam and I had been classmates in graduate school at Cornell University in upstate New York. In fact, we shared the same small laboratory room, it's shelves and tables crowded with abandoned apparatus and junk we'd both devised in our efforts to complete our research and earn our graduate degrees.

When Sam was sick or on vacation, I'd feed his hundreds of hungry adult mosquitoes by inserting my forearm into their big screened cage for a half-hour every other day.

In an odd sort of way, I suppose that made us blood brothers. Conversely, for his part, in a pinch, he'd tend my colonies of lab-raised snails.

We grew to share the same philosophy regarding tropical disease control. We both wished to find ways to stop the spread of diseases such as malaria and snail fever without inflicting severe damage to the environment.

In flight, 12 June 1958

Sam,

I'll make this quick since we're only about twenty minutes out from Aguilas.

I've spent most of the flight reviewing correspondence between George Barlow, my supervisor at the Parasitic Diseases Section (PDS) in Geneva, and Harlan Palma, head of the Taviran Department of Health. I worked briefly with George in Africa two years ago before he was promoted to assistant chief of the PDS. I suppose that contact explains why I was picked for Tavira. I'll be working directly with Harlan Palma and his staff doing necessary background research, evaluating their control program, and making suggestions for improvements.

Several of the letters George forwarded to me are almost scandalous. Apparently, the PDS consultant I'm replacing, Ota Homma, was summarily kicked out—deported. Judging from bits and pieces here and there in the letters, the Tavirans found Homma rude and officious, especially towards two field hands assigned to do the driving, help load and unload equipment, collect water samples, etc. Homma took to ordering them about so ruthlessly, they soon began, as a little joke, to call him Tía Ota *(Aunt Ota) behind his back. Trouble is, Homma couldn't take a joke. About the third time he overheard them, he exploded—sort of went berserk—broke a dip-net over the back of one of them, cursed the other, left them standing there dumbfounded, drove the truck back alone to Aguilas, and holed up in his hotel room for two days. Of course, Harlan Palma was incensed and George was terribly embarrassed.*

However, at least Palma requested a replacement. That suggests to me that he's either a forgiving soul or desperately needs the help.

I'll have to watch it, though! No doubt, it falls to me to try to overcome Homma's negative legacy. I'm sure Palma will have me in his sights from the instant this plane touches down.

Homma did manage to write two excellent papers about studies he did in villages close to Aguilas and along the seacoast, but he never did get out into the boondocks. George sent me drafts of those papers and asked that I comment on them. Like you and me, Homma was opposed to treating the streams with chemicals to kill the snails. He would have agreed with us that this approach is too destructive to the delicate ecosystem of these small tropical creeks and streams.

In that connection, working with you in Puerto Rico has convinced me that the biggest secrets to transmission of [snail fever] are hiding high in the mountain watersheds of these islands. That's going to be my first approach—to study the high-country creeks and streams and the villages that crowd along their banks. On Tavira, those sites seem to have been pretty much ignored.

Just now I caught a beautiful bird's-eye view of Tavira, stem to stern. The island is shaped like a life raft heading north: high mountains forward; flat as Kansas, aft.

Thanks for the productive exchange of ideas while with you those few brief days in Puerto Rico. I'm convinced that your own research is on the right track. In fact, I'll make that clear in several ways in my report to

Geneva. And special thanks for entrusting me with one of your fantastic filtration gadgets. I'll put it to good use. Count on it.

Well, my seat partner says we'll be landing in a few minutes. I must stop. Take care!

Harvey

P.S. - My new address: Harvey Shoals, Hotel Mar Chiquita, Calle Castaños, Aguilas, Tavira

I've bracketed *snail fever* in the fourth to last paragraph of the letter above. In the actual letter, I referred to snail fever as *schisto*, a nickname for *schistosomiasis*, one of the correct names for this deadly disease. In the 1950s, schisto killed well over a million people a year and destroyed the economy of a dozen nations. The death rate is still way up there. Of all the infectious tropical diseases, only malaria kills more humans each year.

I had gathered up my papers and stowed them in my briefcase just as the engines throttled down and the landing-gear winches began to whine. The plane shuddered as the wheels locked into place. The sea appeared placid. The runway at Aguilas was coming up fast.

The plane had two seats on either side of the aisle. I had a window seat on the left side, at about the middle just behind the wing. The big man occupying every scrap of the aisle seat next to me braced his outstretched arms against the back of the headrest in front of him. He peered at me over bulging biceps, grinned, and said, "Best hold on to your hat. Likely land the same way as last week, the week before, and the week before that. There's forty, fifty, pilots flying these cattle-cars somewhere in God's world. Most can land 'em pretty good. This guy's a notorious exception."

My seatmate had a wonderfully engaging smile and a hesitant, yet not unpleasant baritone voice. I was trying to think of something appropriate to say when he spoke again.

"Easier than the old Boeing 247. That one had them two 550-horsepower Pratt and Whitney radial piston Wasp engines. No where near as much pitch control to the propellers."

He appeared to be about fifty, but with a shock of prematurely white hair that nearly covered his ears and extended down over the back of the collar of his short-sleeved, flowered, nylon sport shirt. Similar white hair curled up from a sunburned chest at the level of his collarbone.

The plane hit the runway and bounced. The tires screeched. On the third touchdown the engines roared and the fuselage shook like a wet birddog. Up front, an overhead compartment burst open, dumping pillows, boxes, and shopping bags onto the heads below.

"Flies like my World War II buddy, Howie," the big man said, as the plane bumped past a lineup of fire trucks and ambulances. Sirens screamed as the entire entourage of emergency vehicles took up the chase.

"What's happened," I asked.

"Nothing. The locals expect every landing he makes to be his last. There's a touch of fatalism to the Taviran mindset. You'll get used to it if you stay around long enough."

I turned to study him. He'd used the words *stay around* in an oddly exaggerated way. We'd hardly exchanged a word during the flight. He was obviously a fellow *americano*, and one of my favorite varieties, the kind that employs poor grammar as a tool, turning it on and off at will. The best of them use it with the skill of an analyst to quickly identify insufferable snobs, to judge a stranger's affluence, and perhaps even to guess a person's level of education.

"You a college professor?" he asked. "Don't mean to pry; noticed your slide-rule. California company made mine; looks like real ivory. Fact is, they're a fat goose better than paper an' pencil, but they can't hold a candle to them big new mechanical calculators. Just bought one in San Juan. It's stowed with the baggage. Weighs a bloody ton."

"I'm acquainted with those," I said. I chose not to mention that they had one in the office of the research station in Tanzania—Tanganyika back then. I didn't want to get into that with him. "You'll have fun with it," I added.

"I surely will," he said, looking past me out the window. He wore a pair of seersucker-style nylon trousers—the kind with the pale blue pinstripes. Paper-thin. Cool, no doubt, but they looked dreadful on him. Their seams were stretched the limit.

"Noticed on your briefcase your name's Harvey Shoals. I had a cousin named Shoals; lived in Tacoma; shot down over Schweinfurt; the big raid in October '43. My name's Charlie Bauer, by the way."

He crossed his right arm over the left and we shook hands. "Was you in the army?" he asked.

"Infantry; Pacific," I said. "I was wounded when we retook Manila in February of '45. They shipped me to Leyte and flew me home from there."

"You must have been hit pretty bad."

"Yes." I wanted off the subject. I explained quickly that WHO had just assigned me to Tavira; that I expected to be staying on the island possibly two years.

"*Who?*" he roared.

"I'm sorry," I said. "I dislike acronyms, too. WHO stands for World Health Organization."

Instantly, he seemed to come to attention, as though something rang a bell. "Aha! So you're the new bug doctor! I figured as much from the stuff you've been reading. Then, abruptly, his arms came down and he pulled at a bag under the seat in front of him. "Oops!" he said. "Time to move out."

The plane was still coasting. Charlie Bauer—let me call him *Charlie* since I'm more used to that—Charlie muscled himself free from the hug of the armrests and balanced his great weight on the aisle-side arm of his seat. He said a few more things and then ended the encounter with, "Nice talking with you, Doc. You'll see my name on a lineup of warehouses near the wharf. I'm there day and night. Live upstairs in the middle building. Wife's dead. Might as well warehouse myself along with her furniture. Can't seem to throw it out. Cheap quarters." Then he ended our visit on a more serious note. "If you ever need help, any kind of help, don't hang back. From what I gather, you *could* need help, more of it than you can imagine!"

Obviously, he'd garnered something about me by reading over my shoulder during the flight. Not that it mattered. Most of my papers were just dry letters and research articles, and except for the stuff about Homma, they were businesslike and uninteresting.

More of it than you can imagine! The remark seemed out of place, almost as though he intended to upset me. Why would he want to do that?

By contrast, I had learned little or nothing about him—only that he'd had a friend from Tacoma who was killed or captured during WWII, that he lived alone in one of his own warehouses, and that he'd just purchased a mechanical calculator. Presumably, he was some sort of importer.

He was on his feet and four rows down the aisle before I felt the wedge of hot air that signaled opening of the hatch near the front of the plane. I watched him push his way to the opening, towering above others who were standing, not waiting for them to take their turn to step into the aisle ahead of him.

He was tall, at least six-feet-six. Nothing about him detracted from the obvious first impression that he was from the States. I, myself, was just over six feet, but I was no match for his weight and obvious strength.

Moments later, as I waited in the aisle, a fidgety small boy, apparently the ward of two middle-aged men, crowded up against me. The men were talking rapidly in the soft consonants of Caribbean Spanish. Only a word or two made sense. The boy addressed one of the men in Spanish as Uncle Felix and the taller of the two told him to hush.

I recall vividly the intense heat reflected off the concrete as I stood beside the plane waiting for my luggage to emerge from the baggage compartment. The runway, bleached bone-white by the tropical sun, paralleled a wide strip of yellow sand that sloped gradually down to the surf.

The flight had arrived about half past four in the afternoon. Already, a crimson sky to the west was beginning to suggest a promising tomorrow. Far to the north, the impressive *Montaña Espoleta* reached up beneath an ominous black cloud. The *Espoleta*, "the wishbone," covers the upper fifth of the island, highest like the prow of a ship at the northernmost tip where it meets the sea, and with arms extending southward along both the northeast and northwest coastlines.

I recall catching a faint scent of hibiscus mixed with the odor of aviation fuel. I knew hibiscus well from tropical Africa and Puerto Rico. When I left Tanzania just a few months earlier, tensions were mounting, and I recall that it seemed good to be back in the benign political climate of the Caribbean. As I think back on that moment in my youth, I can't believe that I could have been so totally ignorant of the political strife underway at that moment on Tavira.

I suppose I could say *on Tavira* or *in Tavira*. There seems to be a division point depending on the size of an island. You don't often hear *on Cuba,* but you do often hear *on Saint Thomas*, or *on Saint Lucia*. I wished my command of Spanish were better. I had convinced myself over the years that I had no talent for foreign languages. In college I studied German, which was thought necessary at the time for a major in the sciences. To this day, my mind plays the annoying trick of mixing what few Spanish words I know with a smattering of the German that I remember.

While working with Sam in Puerto Rico I found I could more or less communicate with the villagers in the tiny communities along the rivers and streams surrounding the sugar cane *centrales*. In Puerto Rico, I was never embarrassed talking with rural folks. They were always patient and helpful, and kept listening and questioning until they understood what it was I was trying to explain. However, the pedestrians in San Juan or Rio Piedras or Ponce seemed far less tolerant of my deficiency.

As I crossed the concrete on the way to the terminal building, I noticed a clump of coconut palms near the western end of the building. Except for the palms, the hibiscus, and a few strands of tan grass between cracks in the concrete near where I walked, there was little other vegetation adorning the airport grounds. An apron of concrete extended north on either side of the terminal to sheet-metal hangers. Somewhere north of the hangers was the city of Aguilas, population approximately twenty thousand at the time, about the size of its namesake on the southeastern coast of Spain.

Charlie had already disappeared into the terminal. Through the glass doors, I could see lines forming for customs inspection inside. Somewhere beyond Customs, Luis Barbero of the Taviran Department of Health would be waiting to greet me.

When I reached the lines I set my bag on the tile floor and put the box containing Sam's filtration device beside it.

I kept hold of my briefcase. The line for visitors moved slowly. I shifted the luggage forward with a foot.

The uniformed customs officer who examined my passport asked in perfect English if I would be driving a car while on the island.

"Yes," I said.

"U.S. driver's license?"

I reached for my wallet. "Oh my Gosh!"

The man stared at me through amber glasses and waited. His long, beaklike face, especially with the glasses, conveyed to my mind the impression of a praying mantis ready to strike. "It's gone," I said.

"*Problema*?" the mantis grinned.

"Someone got my wallet. I had it on the plane." I looked around. Charlie was just exiting the building to the street. It couldn't have been Charlie. The wallet was in my left back pocket, the window side. I hadn't left my seat on the short flight.

The two men and the boy had cleared the customs line for returning residents seconds before I entered the visitors' lineup. They, like Charlie, were about to leave the building. "Maybe when I got up to leave the plane . . . There were people crowding along behind me and—"

"There always are," the mantis said. He turned quickly and snapped his fingers at an armed guard watching the inspection area. I noticed that the guard turned and headed for the exit door. "We will disregard about the license. You have a license, yes?"

"Yes. At least I *had* one. I can't believe I—"

"It happens," the customs officer said. "I am sorry. In fact it happens too often lately." Briefly, he removed his glasses. He mopped his sharp features with a handkerchief. "Would you say—off the record, of course—that there is anything of a sensitive nature about this research you plan to do here?" He paused before going on. "I am acquainted with Luis Barbero, the man you are to meet. I'm not suggesting anything, you understand, but do not mention to Luis that I inquired."

"I don't see any way my work could be classed as *sensitive,*" I said. Then I reemphasized, "There was a boy and also two men behind me in the aisle on the plane—"

The mantis cut me off. The passengers in line were restless and inching forward across the wait line. "You are free to go, *señor* Shoals. Not to worry. We will look into this business of your wallet. We have more ways than perhaps you imagine. We are already aware of the two men that you refer to."

"Thanks," I said, taking a quick breath before lifting my heavy bag and the box containing Sam's device. The box was bulky, but not nearly as heavy as the suitcase. The mantis hadn't shown the slightest interest in my possessions.

Luis Barbero, a tall, thin man who moved with a long stride, came towards me from the far side of the terminal. We shook hands and headed for the exit.

Outside at the curb, I mentioned the wallet heist.

"It could have been a random hit with no significance behind it," he said. "But, lately, certain interests alien to the government are known to be using pickpocket experts on the incoming planes, etcetera."

"But why me?" I was grateful that Luis had such a good command of English.

"Presumably because they expect you will be working out in the villages as did your predecessor. I am just guessing, but because *el señor* Ota Homma was here for such a short time, they could easily have considered his ousting as some sort of a ploy to switch him for a secret agent, etcetera."

I wondered if he threw in those *etceteras* when speaking in Spanish, or just when speaking in English. It was disconcerting not to know what more he might have said in place of *etcetera*. And I still didn't get the connection. "Whom do you categorize as *they*?" I asked.

He avoided the question. Instead, he pulled out a crumpled pack of cigarettes. "Care for a smoke?"

"No, thanks," I said. "I don't smoke."

"You are so short for an *americano*, I figured maybe you smoked in your youth and it stunted your growth."

He had to be kidding. We were almost exactly the same height. I considered laughing but chose not to. I wanted to see where he was going with that.

He lit the cigarette, studied my expression, and said, without a trace of a smile, "Just a joke." He was quiet for a moment, then added, "I should quit. Pressures of the job, I suppose."

I wondered, as I settled beside him in the back seat of his chauffeured limousine, how there could be pressures of any consequence working in a paradise no bigger than a postage stamp. Tavira measured less than four hundred square miles, a tenth the size of Puerto Rico. Although densely populated in the small cities, a substantial number of rural sugar cane workers lived along the rivers and streams. But it seemed to me that with such things as citrus, breadfruit, and avocados growing wild by the truckload as they were in Puerto Rico, certainly there could be no shortage of food.

I knew that Tavira had just one sugar cane company, *Centrale Allende*. Luis reminded me that the current president, Juan Bucareli, owned *Centrale Allende*. Back then, in a sugar cane based economy, the breadwinners of almost all rural families worked either in the cane fields or at the *centrale*. Their work was hard and the pay was poor, and like the depression era coal miners of Kentucky and West Virginia, they were constantly in debt to the "company store" at the *centrale*. A worker's pay rarely covered the week's essentials.

Luis's reference to "certain interests alien to the government" continued to concern me. Of course I knew that patterns of poverty such as this one exist in every developing nation. That's what the concept behind the PDS was all about. In countries overburdened by tropical disease, disease control had to come before economic change could be effective.

I knew that leprosy and yellow fever had been wiped out thirty or more years ago. "Do you still have a TB sanatorium?" I asked.

"Yes. We converted part of the old leprosy compound at Corejo for TB. They do good work. Not much of a problem anymore."

"Malaria?"

"Not really. A few suspected cases back in one mountain village last August. I'm not sure we even confirmed them. The mayor requisitioned a supply of quinine. That's all we know."

His indifference to the possible presence of malaria back in the mountains struck me as odd. "Dengue?" I asked.

"Plenty! We don't advertise it. Why should we? Puerto Rico has lots of dengue and they don't advertise it. The *turistas* to Puerto Rico who get it probably never know what hit them. They convalesce back home in Chicago or New York where their doctors chalk it up to some sort of influenza. Regretfully, we do not enjoy so many *turistas* as Puerto Rico. Under the circumstances, do you think our government would advertise the presence of dengue here?"

Odd the way he had gone on about that. I wondered why. "Strange," I said, "the way mosquito-borne diseases seem to hold on so tenaciously."

"Yes it is."

"Which would you rather work on: a waterborne disease like schisto, transmitted by snails; or a mosquito-borne disease like malaria or dengue?"

In the Caribbean form of schisto, the adult worms, called *blood flukes,* live in human blood vessels surrounding the intestine. Their spiny eggs work their way into the intestine. The eggs almost invariably end up in the rivers and streams. In an economy such as Tavira's, the waterways are polluted daily by infected workers returning from the cane fields and by infected school children playing under the foot bridges on the way home from school.

Once in freshwater, the eggs mature and hatch and the larvae invade snails. Some weeks later, from each snail there emerge thousands of a larval form called a *cercaria* that can swim, attach to, and penetrate human skin much as hookworm larvae used to penetrate the feet of barefoot children of the American south up until the late thirties.

Luis answered my question. "I've put in a lot of years on both diseases," he said. "I understand malaria better than schisto. I guess I like to work with what I know. We have a good knowledge of mosquito ecology. We know little about snail populations. I think they are hard to study? Do you agree? I suppose I have an aversion to the unknown."

"How do you mean *aversion to the unknown*? Do you feel you are not making enough progress? You are in charge of the snail studies, I thought?"

"At this time, no *señor*. The very same day that we put Ota Homma on the plane, when I returned from the airport, Doctor Palma moved me from field studies to chemical control."

"Oh for God sake! And Palma thinks he has enough basic information to succeed with chemically killing the snails."

"Exactly! He expects it to work if he can get a big enough spray program underway."

"So that's your assignment?" What a blow this news was to me. I'd been sent to Tavira to help them find an environmentally sound way to limit transmission of the disease. All over the world they had tried killing snails with chemicals without much success. They'd spray the streams; the snails would return; they'd spray again. It was a never-ending, absolutely futile approach.

"Well," I said, somewhat sarcastically, "at least you won't have to worry about the security of your job."

"You are very perceptive, *señor*. With leprosy, TB, and yellow fever gone, schisto is what is left. I must work on what there is to work on. I suppose I should be content if it keeps me occupied until retirement."

I looked at him more closely. I guessed he might be approaching sixty. "But you don't believe it will work?" I said.

"No, it is destined to fail."

"Have you told Palma how you feel about it?"

"Schisto is the devil's own creation," he said. "No matter how they try to control it in different countries, they seem to cause a worse problem of another kind in its place."

It was an oblique answer. I wasn't surprised to learn that he was well informed. He'd been in health work all his life. Obviously, he had an inquiring mind. I listened with interest to the quality of his English, paying attention to his thought processes. He seemed to enjoy formatting an answer that spoke to the question from several points of view.

I hadn't expected the conversation to take this twist so early in our relationship, and I wondered if he was trying to warn me of further disclosures that I needed to prepare myself for.

I felt at home with Luis almost from the moment we first shook hands. An unusual man, tall as me but stoop-shouldered, with a greyhound's head and a lower jaw that seemed more or less permanently unhinged revealing a full complement of huge teeth, he seemed a comfortable person to be with. If there had been enough flesh on his bones to interest even a horsefly, if he'd stood tall, and if he'd displayed a bit more confidence, his bearing would have been impressive and authoritative. Still, he seemed fatherly, sincere, and by no means threatening.

He lit up another cigarette and reminded the driver to pull in at the Hotel Mar Chiquita. "Better think through what you had in that wallet that might give the crooks something they could use—bank account numbers, that sort of thing."

"Good suggestion! Thanks," I said. I scanned the entrance to the hotel. "So this is to be home for the next two years." The chauffeur opened the car door and lifted out my luggage. As we parted, Luis suggested we meet in the lobby of the Department of Health at about nine in the morning. I thanked him for being at the airport.

"*De nada*," he said.

From the curb, I watched the limo merge into the sparse traffic of Aguilas before lifting my luggage and walking to the registration desk of the hotel.

JUNCOS

The Hotel Mar Chiquita reminded me of the quaint hotel on the square in New Orleans where Maggie and I had stayed during our honeymoon trip in December 1941, just days after Pearl Harbor. That one, too, had classical Spanish ironwork on the balconies and heavy furnishings set about its spacious rooms. We were both eighteen, and married in haste before I enlisted.

In college after the war, we lived in recycled army barracks near the campus that were reserved for married veterans. We both completed college—I with the help of the GI Bill, Maggie with financial assistance from her family. She majored in English and dreamed of becoming a successful author. We married far too young, without considering how our career goals might or might not mesh.

During graduate school, I obtained a research assistantship that paid for our basic needs. However, those four years placed a serious strain on our marriage. We both sensed the growing divergence in our ambitions. She was happier and more at peace with herself when she remained at home while I was off on assignment.

We thought we'd solved the problem by setting up housekeeping on a small farm in Towhee, North Carolina, hoping it could become a home base where I could return between consulting assignments. She was extremely happy there, content to participate in community activities, keep her journals, and pursue her writing. On those all-too-brief vacations when I was home on leave, usually in the fall of the year, I'd spent my days splitting firewood to warm the house in winter. We'd walk the woods together in search of wild mushrooms, or climb the trail to clear the newly-fallen leaves from the mountain spring. We had gravity water—water from a spring uphill that required no pump to maintain pressure at the house. We also used kerosene lanterns and candles in lieu of electricity. That was Maggie's choice. She loved the plainness, perhaps the minimalism, of her life at Towhee more than anything else the world could offer.

Maggie loved her austere life so much that she etched the lines of Robert Frost's brief poem, "The Pasture" into a sanded and polished slab of heartwood from a giant red oak, and mounted it on the wall above her kitchen sink. In a way, I think the poem expressed for her the desire that I might grow to share the simple joys she drew from living there, especially in our later years as my consulting work scaled down.

Once, and only once, we'd contemplated divorce. She wanted me to be free to find other relationships more suitable to my personality. I loved her too much to yield to that.

Tragedy took her life during my first year in Tanzania. She died alone in the house of a heart attack, they said. She was thirty-three with no history of heart disease, although we would not have known that anyway since she rarely went for checkups. A neighbor found her several days later. I flew home. I hadn't the courage to put the property up for sale. I locked up the house and asked a Realtor friend in Towhee to look in on things from time to time.

I missed her desperately at first, but my guilt and grief eased as I came to understand from reading her journals the wealth of happiness that filled her days there. I continued to return to Towhee throughout my career whenever vacation time accrued, and I live there now, alone.

The upholstery on the furniture in Room 212 was far from clean, and the salt air had taken its toll. The south wall was partially bricked-up, the bricks and mortar lathered with cheap plaster and paint, repair work following a fire perhaps, or crude in-house remodeling. The room had a private bath, but the paint on the ceiling in the shower was peeling away in shards the size of potato chips.

I had just removed my shirt to shave before dinner when there was a knock at the door.

"*Momentito*!" I called.

As I opened the door a police badge caught my attention. "Now what?" I asked.

"*Señor*," the officer said, "your wallet." He held it out in the palm of his hand as though he'd just picked it off the hallway carpet.

"Well, I'll be damned!" I took it from him and turned it over in my hands. It seemed intact. At least it had not been stripped of its contents. "So where did you find it?"

He ignored the question. "Please examine the contents and tell us what is missing. We will try to make good any loses and assist you in replacing important papers and travelers checks, if any have been taken."

I examined the wallet more carefully. Five crisp U.S. hundred-dollar bills did not belong to me. But the approximately four hundred dollars in smaller denominations—all the money that I was carrying—was gone. "There's more money here than I started with," I said.

"We thought so."

"How come?"

"It happens. We do not know why."

"Thanks. I appreciate your bringing it around."

Without a word, the officer gave a casual salute and turned towards the elevator. I closed and locked the door. I went back a moment later and attached the chain as well. I also checked the window and the door to the balcony. I wasn't keen on being robbed a second time.

Breakfast the next morning at the Mar Chiquita was quite adequate and came with the price of the room. However, I was too much on edge to enjoy it. I settled for hot oatmeal and coffee. The scrambled eggs on a tablemate's plate looked okay, but his toast came soaked with melted butter. My three tablemates were salesmen from the States, two were marketing crop insecticides; the other, pharmaceutical drugs. I was running late and pretty much ignored them.

I walked to the Department of Health. It was only four short blocks from the hotel.

Luis Barbero was waiting in the lobby. "So you managed to survive the night?"

"I did. And I'm all the more wealthy for it, too."

"Meaning what, exactly?"

"The police returned my wallet."

"I'm glad. Not empty?"

I started to tell him of the five hundred dollars, but thought better of it. "Not at all. Very little missing."

"Then I am especially happy for you. Happy for a successful conclusion to the wallet episode. It would have made a poor introduction to Tavira to begin by chasing after all the many things you lose when you lose a wallet."

After a moment, he added, "Well, what is your pleasure?"

"I want to get out into the countryside. I want to look at those mountains. Are there any roads up into the *Montaña Espoleta*?"

"That I cannot answer. There used to be. However, it has been years since I have ventured into the *Espoleta*. I can send you out with Salvador García. It would take all day. Or, if you prefer, you can spend the morning in our library reviewing our recent pathetic efforts to control the disease . . . You can also suggest that we ignore both options and spend the day at the beach. Your predecessor would have chosen the beach. My advice would be not to emulate him. Therefore, I have asked Salvador not to leave for the field until you have a chance to decide."

I was intrigued with his oblique reference to Ota Homma, and the warning not to emulate him, but I decided to let that lie.

"Tell me about Salvador García," I said.

"Elderly," he said without expression. "Lives in the village of Juncos about fifteen miles north at the base of the mountains. He knows the countryside and he knows schisto. A visit to Juncos would be a good introduction."

"Agreed," I said. "The library can wait till tomorrow."

"Harlan Palma wants to talk with you. But that, too, must wait. He is tied up today."

"Frankly, I'm glad of that. Not very tactful of me, but it's the truth. I'm more eager to get my hands into things."

Luis seemed to study me thoughtfully. Then he said, "May I ask you to tell me again something about where you have worked, etcetera?"

"Yes, of course. I've just come from working briefly in Puerto Rico. We found literally dozens of places where people become infected—almost entirely where small streams flow through the little villages where the sugar cane workers live."

"I believe you mentioned Tanganyika?"

He was referring to Tanzania by its previous name. "Yes. As recently as this spring. I was there two years."

"And you mentioned South Africa?"

I paused. "No, I don't believe I did."

"Then I must have read that in your file. They always send a file, you know."

My interest in Luis sharpened. I had spent a brief time at the research station at Nelspruit before flying north to Tanzania. It surprised me to learn that Luis had the opportunity to size me up even before we met. I was grateful that he seemed friendly and with no sign of prejudgment. I mentioned a couple of things that were different about schisto in Africa.

Luis interrupted. "Do you see the skinny fellow by the cigarette machine?"

"Yes."

"That is Salvador. Do not expect him to understand much English. He is a good driver. He knows every road and village between here and the *Espoleta.*

"However, do not underestimate him or talk down to him. That is the best advice I can give you. Have you ever noticed how some people will exaggerate their pronunciation and speak louder than usual when they talk to an obviously handicapped person? I've seen them do that with uneducated persons, too. I beg you never to do that. I like you, *señor* Shoals. I think you can do us some good. However, if you are to succeed here in your work, the rural people must also like you, and they must grow to trust you."

Obviously, Luis was not going to let go of the Homma incident without speaking his mind. I figured I'd eventually learn more than I wanted to know about that. Nevertheless, I felt a measure of relief to have apparently passed his preliminary examination.

Strangely, his sudden familiarity ceased as quickly as it had begun. "You have been assigned an International Scout with 4-wheel drive. Salvador is accustomed to it and you might as well let him do most of the driving."

"Sounds good."

"Salvador will have hip boots, dip-nets, and the other usual paraphernalia in the Scout. I suggest you test the boots for leaks before you rely on them. You must understand that the locals have lived with schisto all their lives. They find it difficult to worry about a bit of river water the way you and I might. He will also have plenty of isopropyl alcohol for your hands. Few workers here use rubber gloves. We cannot get them to wear them. Too hot. On the other hand, we *have* taught them to apply alcohol when they accidentally get their hands wet.

"Yet, you watch. They will pick snails out of a dip-net with their bare fingers. Most dangerous thing they could do. Never think to sterilize their hands with alcohol after they do it."

He paused and seemed to be thinking of something else. Then he said, "You should not interpret Salvador's assignment to you as a compliment. Believe me! Two years ago, Palma assigned him to me. He's stubborn as a mule, twice as independent, and unquestionably as smart. Think of him as God's gift to ensure the survival of schisto on Tavira. This is because just when you think you have everything going right, everything will suddenly go wrong."

I had to laugh. "From what you say, it appears that Salvador and I are two of a kind."

He glanced at me briefly and said, "I'd hold that conclusion somewhat in abeyance if I were you."

Many of the comments that Luis made over the following weeks as I got to know him better—side comments about the Department, his co-workers, and government in general—were obviously intended in jest. However, his was a brand of humor quite definitely on the mordant side. I soon learned that he was the superlative straight man, and during the eighteen months that I worked with him, just once did I see so much as a hint of a smile.

"Ah, he sees you," Luis said, nodding towards the cigarette machine. "I will leave you two to work things out. We can talk later." With that, he dexterously caught a closing elevator door with an enormously long arm, stepped inside, and disappeared.

By contrast to Luis, Salvador had a smile that could win an election. And apparently he already had, I soon learned.

I extended a hand. "Harvey Shoals."

"*Sí, doctor.* I am Salvador." The little man spoke with a strong voice that rasped over every word. Yet, he did not offer his hand in return.

"Luis Barbero suggested I ride with you today."

"*Sí* . . . Juncos," Salvador said, and the smile broadened.

"I'm ready whenever you are."

"*Sí, doctor. Vámonos!*" Then after a pause, "Juncos is my home, *doctor*."

"Yes, so Luis said."

"*Sí*." Salvador continued to stand, the broad smile unchanged.

I gave a quick nod that finally got him moving.

Salvador was less than five-feet-six—perhaps five-three or four. He was so thin that his khaki trousers hung in folds about his hips. The trousers and his worn and sweat-stained khaki shirt were WWII vintage. Luis had inferred that he had some age on him. His face was as lined and rough as water-buffalo hide, and about the same slate-gray cast. The smooth, raven-blackness of youth appeared dusted with the potash and lime of a hundred plantings and harvests. This man had to be in his late seventies or even past eighty.

As we drove off in the Scout, and as he coped with the Aguilas traffic, I asked him his age. He admitted that he wasn't certain of his birth date. However, he remembered events that had occurred during his childhood and youth. Eventually, together, we concluded that he must have been born sometime during 1878 or 1877, which would make him eighty or eighty-one.

The exercise intrigued me. Here was a man who had learned more English than I had Spanish, and a man whose mind could sift through facts with skill and accuracy. I knew from that instant I would like him.

The Scout was far from new. The odometer had logged over seventy thousand miles. But I was glad to have the use of it. Sam used one in Puerto Rico and swore by it for reliability in rough terrain.

"Have you lived in Juncos a long time?"

"All my life, *doctor.*"

"Born there?"

"*Sí*. Born there."

"Is it better to live in Juncos than Aguilas?"

"*Doctor*, you know what happen? I am mayor of Juncos. *Sí*, Juncos is a good place to live."

Salvador's question, *Doctor, you know what happen*, caught me off guard. Apparently, it was his way of introducing a thought slightly more complicated than a simple *yes* or *no,* and in such a way as to give him time to phrase a thought in English.

It occurred to me that Salvador wanted me to know he had responsibilities apart from his job with the Department of Health. I thought of asking what sort of problems he dealt with as mayor of an upland village, but I began to notice that the strain of getting acquainted seemed to be distracting him from his driving. I resolved to let him initiate any new conversation.

In the silence that ensued, I mused that I was similarly handicapped. I often found myself unable to study a microscope slide while talking, or review research data while eating. No doubt I focused too completely on whatever task was at hand. Salvador and I seemed to share that trait.

Once away from the coast and into the rolling wooded countryside, Salvador approached every blind curve with a blast of the car horn and hugged the right side of the road. Our route snaked north beside shallow streams were, just as in Puerto Rico, women slapped balled clothing against smooth stones, while naked children splashed happily in pools of sun-warmed water. Occasionally, we passed close to a muddy oxbow of a creek where a tethered pig wallowed in the wet mud and sent spurs of murky water coursing downstream.

We crossed a row of steep foothills, returned to flat plain, then drove through three or four inches of water across the gravel shallows of the broad *Rio Ebro* to reach its northern side. Salvador explained that we could only come this way during the dry season when the *Ebro* was low. During the wet season, or when the river was running high from rains, we would have to use the bridge in Comerio much further east. That would add a half-hour to the trip each direction.

After fording the *Ebro*, Salvador turned west on a dirt and gravel road that followed the north bank of the river.

It was near noon when we reached Juncos and parked the Scout in the solid shade of a broad-leafed African tulip tree. Contrary to what I expected, Juncos was not a town at all. There were no stores or public buildings. It was only a typical sugar cane worker's village consisting of several dozen tin-roofed shanties perched on stilts.

Close to where we parked, a small creek named the *Quebrada Perico*, joins the *Ebro* on its way to the sea. At the confluence of these two, the waters of the little *Perico* flow out in a translucent arc for ten or fifteen feet before merging completely into the overwhelming volume of the muddy *Ebro*.

The best constructed of the homes seemed to be those closest to the edge of the *Perico*. All were spaced out at regular intervals, with perhaps fifty feet between. Homes further from the water and further up into the forest were generally smaller and not as well built. Yet, they had greater privacy and better shade located as they were among the trees. Dirt paths worn deep into the hillsides crisscrossed between them, so that a virtual spider web of trails enjoined every house to every other in the community.

Beneath the tulip tree, the Scout's tires rested on a smooth, dry, gravel wash created probably not so much by floodwaters of the *Ebro* as by the *Perico* itself as the runoff from heavy rains swept the gravel down from the rain forest above. If Juncos were farther from the mountain, sand or gravel of a smaller size might have covered the banks of the stream. However, Juncos stood right up against the lofty terrain of the *Espoleta*.

From our vantage point close to the confluence of this diminutive stream and the *Ebro*, we could look out across the river to the south to acre after acre of sugar cane fields, extending for several miles at least. Downriver to the west and about a mile away, also on the north side of the *Ebro*, *Centrale Allende* stood tight against a sheer cliff. The *centrale's* massive smoke stack, silhouetted against the face of the cliff, reached at least a hundred feet above the huge boilers used to produce raw sugar from great mounds of crushed cane.

There were no cars at Juncos. The only road to the village, hardly more than a wagon trail, was the one we had just used to reach Juncos after crossing the shallows of the *Ebro*. To the west, this primitive road ended where we parked. To the east, this same road led all the way to Comerio, the nearest town of any size.

Kids of all ages soon crowded about the Scout curious to know who their mayor had brought to visit, and why.

"*Doctor*, you know what happen? They think you *el doctor* Palma. They know *el doctor* Palma is my boss and *el doctor* Palma is boss of Luis. I explain to them another day."

I looked around amongst the houses. "Where do you buy food?"

"*La centrale*," Salvador said.

"The men walk to work at *la centrale*?"

"*Sí*. Always walk."

"There is no connecting road between Juncos and *la centrale?*" I could see traces of a well-worn path on the other side of the *Perico*.

"*Nada*. Must walk." He had noticed that I'd seen the path.

"How do children get to school?"

"*La guagua*, the bus, *señor,* to Comerio."

Salvador pointed out his house, upstream perhaps two hundred feet from where we'd parked. I learned that his wife had died many years ago; that he continued to occupy the home he'd built for her; that he usually took his dinner with his daughter, Francesca, who lived in one of the uppermost houses, and whose husband had been killed in a tractor accident several years back.

I also learned that Salvador's grandson, Hernando, was a senior in high school that year and would enter the agricultural college at Comerio in the fall, and that Salvador was very proud of him as he was of all of his children and grandchildren.

I expressed interest in the fact that Juncos was served by a school bus.

"*Sí*. For last ten years."

"Most of the men work at *la centrale*, I suppose?"

Salvador shrugged. "Or in field. *La zafra*, harvest."

"And how do *you* get to Aguilas to work?"

"Bus. School bus."

"To Comerio? And then I suppose you take another bus to Aguilas?"

"*Sí*."

The kids had wandered off by now. I got out and walked down to the edge of the *Ebro*. I returned to the Scout and rummaged through the equipment in the back until I found a wire dip-net for snails and a glass jar. I walked along several hundred feet of the *Ebro*, dipping into the vegetation at the edge of the river, looking for snails, but found only one or two. I turned to find Salvador at my side with another dip-net and jar. Salvador pointed to the smaller *Quebrada Perico*. I nodded. We both searched the vegetation bordering the stream.

We both found several snails. I filled my jar three quarters full of water and set it in a spot of sunlight on the hood of the Scout. Salvador did the same.

Salvador rolled a cigarette and lit it. He offered it to me. I declined. In a moment or two he lifted his jar and stepped to where he had it in full sunlight. Obviously, he knew what we expected to find. "*Doctor. Mucho cercariae! Mucho!*"

That Salvador knew the technical name for the larval stage that invades the skin of humans caught me by surprise. I should not have been surprised. This diminutive old man had lived and worked with schisto far longer than I. His oversized, olive drab, WWII fatigues were as deceiving as his whiskered face and weathered features. No doubt the accumulated insight of this aging field assistant ran deeper than my textbooks ever could.

I took the jar from him, got the sun on it, and squinted to sharpen my focus. Like tiny silver daggers, hundreds, perhaps a thousand cercariae flickered their way towards the surface and then drifting back down, enough in that one glass to kill a dozen children previously unexposed. With the unaided eye I could barely make out the beating forked tails that enhance their movements and distinguish them from a host of similar species.

Observing cercariae in a jar always calls to mind those dime store, liquid-filled, glass paperweights that you shake and then watch the shimmering particles gradually settle.

Cercariae are active swimmers and live for many hours after their release from the snails. Always suspended, always rising then drifting down, then rising once again, they seem never to tire. During this short phase of their complex life cycle, they search their new environment for a warm leg or an arm to invade. Penetration of human skin takes but a moment. Once they reach the protection of the underlying connective tissue, they rest a bit before continuing their migration to the veins of the intestine of their host.

In my excitement, I went on and on without consideration for Salvador's limited command of English. "I'll want to set up a study area here to get regular counts of the number of snails found and the percentage of snails infected. What I'm after is knowing something of the seasonal frequency of infected snails and the daily variation in the presence of cercariae here at Juncos. This will make a perfect site."

Before I caught myself, I had gone on to say, "We know from the literature that release of the cercariae from the snails is triggered by sunlight. Other than that, we don't really know much about fluctuations in the daily and seasonal presence of the larvae in the rivers and streams."

Salvador seemed to be studying his feet, looking deeply annoyed. Unfortunately, there was no way I could retract my blunder or repeat in Spanish what I'd said. I did my best to apologize. I asked if he knew of other places like this one where we could look for snails. He pointed upstream. I shook my head and waved towards the horizon.

Salvador grinned that marvelous grin. "*Sí, doctor. Muchos*. I show you. *Vámonos!*"

Staff Meeting

Harlan Palma, Director of the Taviran Department of Health, instead of placing me across from him at his huge desk, graciously asked me to sit with him on a comfortable sofa in a quiet alcove of his office where we could look south over the rooftops of the city all the way to the sea. As we waited for his *lieutenants* to join us, we watched the arrival of what was probably the morning flight from San Juan.

Even from where we sat, perhaps two miles from the airport, I could recognize the hopscotch landing and the pursuing rescue vehicles that had inspired Charlie Bauer to ridicule Taviran Airlines.

Doctor Palma asked briefly about my flight and my hotel accommodations. He spoke graciously of his work and his ambition to see his fellow countrymen freed of the tropical diseases that consign them to poverty. He painted for himself a span of formative years growing up in the countryside, familiar with the life and work in the sugar cane fields. The youngest son of a former field supervisor for *Centrale Allende*, he described how he progressed through the ranks to administrative levels within the company. He emphasized how Governor Juan Bucareli, himself, who owned the factory and many acres of the land on the island devoted to sugar cane, and who held his father in high esteem, had personally encouraged him as a sort of mentor; and how, gradually, his interests and goals shifted from the world of business towards the medical needs of his fellow islanders.

Palma was no longer a young man. He was forty before he decided to study medicine. I judged him to be about fifty-five. He was short, but large boned and heavy—most of the extra weight in fat. It seemed hard to imagine him actually doing physical work in the cane fields in his youth even as a supervisor such as his father had been.

In the natural course of events, in view of his family connections, once he had obtained his medical degree, President Bucareli put him in charge of the Department of Health. He had held the position for only six years.

I considered asking him if he was acquainted with Charlie Bauer, but changed my mind. There was something disingenuous about Palma's repeated emphasis on bettering the medical needs of his fellow islanders. Privately, I wondered again the significance of Charlie Bauer's curious offer of help. It wasn't a casual "if I can lend a hand" or "stop by for martinis first chance you get." Distinctly, Charlie had implied *if you find yourself in trouble*.

Palma inquired about the theft of the wallet, exactly how and when I thought it was taken. Again, privately, my thoughts turned to the youngster who had crowded against me as we stood in the aisle waiting to disembark. Had the child actually lifted the wallet, or did he have merely the role of distracter while the more experienced fingers of "Uncle Felix" did the actual purloining. And I wondered what they expected to learn from it once they had it. Would they look for membership cards or other identifying instruments that might define the nature of my visit as Luis had implied? And why did they take the small denomination bills and replace them with crisp hundreds in U.S. currency?

Luis entered the room with one other man whom he introduced to me as Gregorio Ponloja, and with an attractive young woman whom he introduced as Emilia D'Israeli. Palma clarified Gregorio's role as that of departmental financial officer; Emilia, as head of the lab; both as long-term civil servants. They took seats about the alcove.

Luis brought up the wallet heist. They couldn't seem to leave it alone.

"It happens quite often these days," Palma said. The same remark the customs man had made. "No one seems to 'have a handle on it,' as you say in the States. What doesn't make sense is the business of removing the money and then replacing it with hundred dollar bills."

I knew I had not told Luis about the five crisp bills. Hence, Palma may have obtained that information from a police report, some sort of interdepartmental report, or other means. Perhaps he had just assumed it from prior cases.

"It might be some sort of money-laundering scheme," Luis suggested.

"No way," Gregorio said. "There are faster ways to launder money with far less risk."

"Tell us about your trip yesterday with Salvador?" Palma asked, putting an end to the wallet topic.

"Good," I said. "We visited Juncos, found a few infected snails, and then looked at a couple of other sites on the way back to Aguilas."

"Luis will take care of that spot in Juncos immediately. Before the week is out," Palma said, catching Luis's eye.

I was stunned. "No, sir! Please," I said. "We need that as a study area!" I was aghast. The last thing I wanted was to have the *Perico* sprayed with chemicals.

Palma appeared puzzled. "We cannot allow a known transmission site to expose the population to infection on a daily basis just because you want to study it. That is not acceptable," he said. "It would be unethical."

"But Doctor, the problem in schisto control the world over is that we don't know enough about the ecology of the disease. Often the snails, in countries where I've studied them, seem to be transients that appear periodically, then wash on downstream with the first modest rain and are gone. We don't know how long infected snails live in nature. Often, we don't even know where these snail populations breed, or where they become infected, or when dangerous levels of cercariae are present in—"

"You are out of line, *señor*," Palma said. "Your assignment here, as I understand it, is to locate infected areas so that my spray crew can eliminate them. Luis has a spray crew. We expect soon to have many, many crews. We also expect soon to have a great quantity of chemical. We have a commitment to the public to do this."

"I would agree with you wholeheartedly, if that would accomplish anything," I said. "The trouble is, you can kill the snails at a site and they're back within the week. It's a never ending cycle and a costly one. It is the most costly way to attempt to achieve control. We need to study these sites through several seasons. There are important things to learn." I shifted about on the sofa to face Palma directly. "It's not that the chemicals don't kill the snails. They do! But that's a stopgap routine that you'll have to go on repeating for the next hundred years. We can learn to do better than that. All we need is a few months to—"

"Perhaps we had better get this straight here at the start!" Palma said, raising his voice dramatically. "Obviously, you have a vastly different concept of your assignment than I. Now if you believe that I have it wrong, tell me and I will contact your superiors in Geneva and straighten things out! One of us is confused. Perhaps you're not the man for the work we intend to pursue here on Tavira."

For an uncomfortable moment, Palma watched me like a cat with a mouse, obviously letting his statement sink in. Although his size and strength were far from threatening he did not seem a person who could gracefully back down once he'd expressed his position so strongly. Without looking away, he said, "Luis, I'd like you to work closely with Harvey here for a few days until he gets his role well in mind. I want him to have a good orientation to our program so that he steps off on the right foot so to speak. Can you manage that?"

"*Sí, señor!*" Luis said.

It saddened me to note how quickly Luis complied—almost as though he fancied Palma might reprimand him for failing to salute. If only he'd had the guts to say something like, "Well, Harvey may have a point." But I sensed that Palma did not intend to face again the kind of problem he'd encountered with Ota Homma. As far as he was concerned, I was going to be carefully supervised from the start.

I changed the subject and asked Palma what kind of chemical he was using against the snails. Palma fielded the question to Luis. But before Luis could answer, Emilia spoke up. Her command of English seemed excellent. So excellent in fact that I detected something in the choice of her words and in certain inflections in her voice that suggested a desire to distance herself from the others in the room. Neither did she seem to have any trouble stepping up to the plate to answer when her boss was obviously highly irritated.

There was a trace of emotion in her choice of words that only an *americano* such as I might have been likely to detect as she said, "It is the sodium salt of the very most toxic of the chlorophenols. Doctor Palma and others who find acronyms convenient for one reason or another like to refer to it as SCP, and so that is what we have been calling it ever since it first surfaced as the logical solution to all our problems as some of us visualize them." She glanced at me significantly as she added, "We tried *Copper sulfate* in dilute solution, but some argued that it damaged the irrigated sugar cane at certain stages of growth. However, SCP appears to have its own bizarre and subtle characteristics."

I wanted to say, "That's the understatement of the year!" But I guessed correctly that such sarcasm would not sit well with Palma. I knew even back then—perhaps the whole world except Tavira knew back then—that SCP was a ghastly choice. It was no longer used in most countries. It killed every vestige of life in a stream from the insect food that fish depend on, to the fish themselves.

Abruptly, Palma launched into a lengthy defense of SCP that left no doubt that he intended to see a substantial expansion of its use.

I glanced at Emilia as he spoke. She was expressionless. It would be some months before I understood how deeply she distrusted Palma's motivations, both on the intellectual and personal level.

Before that disturbing meeting ended, Palma and I got into several other scraps over related issues: the toxicity of SCP compared to several alternative chemicals; the advantages and limitations of putting the emphasis on community education rather than on chemical treatment of rivers and streams; the total and complete refusal of Palma to allow me to "squander" my time on basic studies of snail ecology and disease transmission.

Throughout this contest of authority, Gregorio, the financial officer, seemed incredibly supportive of Palma. Repeatedly, Luis missed what I considered tactful opportunities to come to my aid. Emilia, alone, seemed consistently more in my camp than did either of the men.

The toxicity of SCP to fish and other stream life was known worldwide in 1958. In addition, a few workers suspected SCP-contaminated water of causing human cancers. There was little firm evidence back then for the cancer claim. However, unexplained spikes in cancer incidence kept cropping up where SCP had been used. It was not until the '70s and '80s that *dioxin*, an impurity in industrial grade SCP, began to be blamed for these cancers.

What a time bomb I seemed to be sitting on. And I'd been on Tavira less than a week!

Even disregarding the cancer claim, I had no doubt that widespread use of the chemical would convert the tropical paradise of Tavira, with its crystalline waterfalls and bubbling streams, into an ugly, silent scene of lethal, gray water tainted with the sickening scent of phenol.

No longer, on quiet tropical evenings, would spirited fish rise to feed on lavish hatches of stonefly nymphs. And on any lazy summer afternoon countless great blue heron, with telltale ruffled plumage, would surely stand rigid awaiting death without the joy of spearing a final dace or darter from amidst the coastal mangroves.

Used in the volume needed to contain the snail population, I felt certain that SCP would challenge Tavira's beauty and win.

As the meeting ended, Palma ordered once more that the *Perico* receive a heavy dose of SCP before the weekend. I had lost a prime study site.

As a final shot at me, Palma ordered Luis to inform Salvador that he was to report to Luis immediately any transmission sites that either of us found. Palma left no doubt that Salvador would be at dire risk of losing his job if he failed to comply.

At the same time, Palma ordered *me* to report directly to *him* all transmission sites that *I* found. I'm sure he figured one of us would entrap the other if we tried to disobey.

I found the obvious intent to convey distrust infuriating, and instantly decided to circumvent him in any way I could.

I left the meeting under a growing cloud of depression. What could I do? I could cable Geneva. However, I felt that approach could come back and bite me. I was on Tavira as the advisor. I wasn't supposed to go crying to Geneva for help. And, anyway, Geneva had no authority to order Palma about. I was there to persuade, not command. Obviously, my mission was off to an incredibly bad start.

DUPLICITY

Within the week, Luis had sprayed enough SCP at Juncos to force the villagers to haul water from a hundred yards upstream in order to avoid the insidious odor and taste of phenol. The daily social event of washing clothes also moved to an upstream site.

I soon discovered that I had a compatriot in Salvador who seemed to have a sixth sense about schisto. From our very first working days together Salvador understood instinctively what I was trying to achieve. Occasionally, he would start a day with his rasping, "*Doctor*, you know what happen? Today we going to find a way." It was uncanny how frequently his prediction would prove true. We would discover a solution to a bewildering problem on the very day he would utter those words.

At eighty, Salvador had lived to see schisto take the lives of many close friends and many of the village children. He was a careful observer with a layman's knowledge of the disease. The ease with which he would adapt to a new experimental approach convinced me that the same idea must have crossed his mind sometime in the past. No subject aroused Salvador's contempt more quickly than did the concept of the widespread use of SCP. In fact, he condemned the use of any chemical, lumping them all together as evil.

As each day with Salvador passed, I came to realize more fully that my helpmate possessed an innate, almost mystical appreciation of the intricate relationship between schisto and his villagers. Without a day's tenure in a classroom he had achieved, at least to my mind, the rank of "pretty-darn-good" epidemiologist.

Salvador was the first and only person on Tavira to tell me, in his halting English, that he believed using SCP aggravated the situation and caused more intense levels of transmission than had existed before its use. I was aware of this phenomenon from other countries where I'd worked. He was overwhelmed with joy when he and I later demonstrated this to be so. However, it was weeks before the two of us felt certain that we knew *why* this was so.

It has always been of profound interest to me that humans living close to the soil have resolved countless complex interrelationships inherent in their environment. I often wonder how many lives it cost Native Americans to learn which mushrooms were lethal, which hallucinogenic, and which could be safely eaten as food.

In Asia, how many batches of the soybean-based *tempeh* caused how many violent outbreaks of enteritis before Asian women learned how to care for the beans during the critical hours while the *Rhizopus* mold multiplied to crowd out the competition from other microbes?

In Georgia and Tennessee, how many batches of pokeweed sickened how many eager foragers before they learned how to prepare and serve that delicious green? Or how much deadly-nightshade root took how many lives before that plant's mother lode of atropine began saving lives?

Natives in South America knew the value of Cinchona bark for treating malaria centuries before researchers identified quinine and quinidine as the active ingredients.

Salvador, in spite of his distress over Luis's repeated chemical applications at Juncos, never blamed Luis directly. Salvador understood what I had just begun to sense: namely, that Luis lacked the courage to push his luck with Palma very far. Had I understood at that early stage what Palma had in mind for Tavira, I'd have been able to accept Luis's timidity more easily, for the scope of Palma's plan left no room for employees who chose not to be team players.

In spite of the damage done to the *Perico* by Luis's spray team, Salvador and I continued to study the *Perico's* watershed. Over the following weeks, we obtained some important data on snail repopulation following the use of that deadly chemical. Each time Luis sprayed, Salvador and I would do careful snail repopulation counts, and we would check to see how many of these new snails were actively releasing cercariae.

While both Salvador and I were admittedly often somewhat tardy about notifying our respective superiors of the return of the snails, as soon as we had stripped from the poisoned stream all the information it could reveal, Salvador would dutifully contact Luis and I would respectfully inform Palma that the snails were back and the stream needed to be retreated. Luis would promptly spray until every snail was surely dead. Then, once again, we'd take up our vigil for the return of infected snails.

While a good, hard, rain would wash snails down from upstream in large numbers, small numbers of snails appeared downstream even in the absence of rain. However, for some curious reason, in the absence of rain, practically every snail that appeared downstream was infected and actively releasing cercariae.

Salvador suggested that infected snails from upstream might lose their hold on the water plants they were attached to more easily than strong, healthy snails. Unlike other freshwater snails, many of which attached their streamlined shells firmly to submerged stones, our snail, *Australorbis glabratus*, resembled a garden slug with a fat nickel stuck upright to its back. As it browsed amongst the submerged plants near the edge of a stream, the clumsy discus shell swung haphazardly about in the changing currents. *Australorbis* was better adapted to aquarium life than to the varying conditions of a mountain stream. If time had been on our side, I believed we might have found a way to put Salvador's theory to a proper test. It was certainly an intriguing observation.

As our understanding of snail repopulation increased, Salvador and I grew eager to study the upper reaches of the *Perico* watershed. Obviously, considering the rapid rate of repopulation, there was plenty to be learned up there in the canyons of the *Espoleta.*

I found it quite unnecessary to warn Salvador not to tell Luis any details about our work at Juncos. Salvador seemed always to be a bit ahead of me on whatever deceptions were needed to thwart Palma's authority. One day at Juncos, after noting my growing depression with Luis's chemical attacks, Salvador said, "*Doctor*, you know what happen? We find many better places than Juncos." And as always, he was true to his word.

During the weeks that followed, as Salvador took me to dozens of productive sites, we would decide which to report to Luis and to Palma and which to keep as study areas just for ourselves. We both agreed to the necessity of reporting *some* sites, just enough to defray suspicion. Hence, for many months, I was able to accomplish a rewarding amount of basic investigation even while finding myself irreparably at odds with Palma, a circumstance that worsened with every passing day.

In the Hands of the Guerrillas

It was about this time that I became better acquainted with Emilia D'Israeli. On several occasions, when I had decided to spend the day in Aguilas, perhaps using the Department of Health library or because I had meetings to attend with Palma or others, Emilia and I would lunch together in the Department cafeteria. Or, if it were not a convenient time for lunch, we went to Rubie's on the opposite side of Calle Castaños for *café con leche*. Rubie steamed the milk and coffee concentrate over a propane flame with the greatest of care, holding the heavy pewter pan by both side-handles and swirling it with the same motion used by her forebears as they panned gold along the banks of the *Rio Ebro*. Eventually, the ingredients, some of them a trade secret, combined to impart a nutlike flavor to the final brew.

One evening, Emilia invited me for dinner at her apartment, which was not at all far from Rubie's on a side street off Calle Castaños. She proved herself a gracious hostess and a talented cook. At home, she appeared somehow smaller and softer than at work, and far less wooden in her responsiveness. I learned from her photographs and stories something of her happy childhood and youth growing up in Comerio, the daughter of one of Tavira's best-loved surgeons. Her mother was a successful attorney. Hence, she had advantages few other children on Tavira could even dream of experiencing.

She talked at length about her undergraduate schooling at Syracuse University in New York State where she also went on to receive her Master of Science degree, specializing in malariology under one of America's true experts in that field.

She was dressed that evening in a delicately flowered shift. About her neck she wore an exquisitely carved short strand of black coral beads that matched the color of the pupils of her eyes. Although she said it was a gift, curiously, when I asked, she sidestepped telling me from whom.

At work, from our first meeting in Palma's office, I had assumed that her woodenness must be some sort of façade contrived to convince Palma that she lacked any vestige of female hormones that Palma might assume would interfere with management of her laboratory staff. However, I was puzzled to find that same aloofness, at least at the outset, in the privacy of her home. In some way or other, at that time, Emilia seemed to me to be withholding information that she felt I was not yet ready to know. I sensed that there was something that she did not care to or dare to reveal. And yet, I also sensed that she was of two minds in this respect. Apparently, at that stage of our relationship she liked me but did not trust me sufficiently to confide in me.

We talked well into the night of her childhood and mine, her ambitions and mine. We had moved to the sofa to share an after-dinner brandy.

Emilia must have read my mind. She stopped her line of thought and said, "You do not get lonely being away from your friends back home for so many long stretches of time?"

"I suppose I do. Yes, occasionally."

"What is her name, Harvey? There must be someone special because you are so special."

"Maggie," I said.

"But that is a nickname, no? For Margaret, perhaps?"

"No. That's her given name, spelled just as it sounds."

"And would she not be appallingly jealous if she could see you now sitting here in the apartment of a young and beautiful woman?"

I laughed. "Accurate Emilia, as always! You are indeed beautiful, Emilia, and in your very own intellectual as well as physical way." She *was* outstanding. Black eyes and black hair accented her pale-white, delicate brow and high cheekbones.

"And your Maggie trusts you in such situations as you find yourself at this moment?"

She had set her brandy glass on the coffee table in front of us. We were sitting very close to each other studying a photo album. Abruptly, she took my hand in both of hers, held it first to her breast, then raised it to her lips and gave a knuckle or two a soft kiss.

"But you are human, too?" she said, as I set my own glass down and took her hands in mine.

Truly, I longed for the intimacy she seemed to be offering. Yet, just as I was about to embrace her, I sensed that this was not for real. Perhaps she drew back ever so slightly. I don't know exactly what small signal I perceived, but something stopped me.

Appropriately, I said, "Well, almost, maybe," referring to her question about being human. "But not in the way you are just now thinking." I smiled openly. It was the sort of statement that would have hurt and angered any lesser woman. Instead, she blushed and then she laughed, and I knew I'd judged her correctly. With some kind of goal in mind, she'd set out to test me and suddenly realized that she had overstepped her own modesty.

"A lucky girl your Maggie," she said.

I didn't tell her then that Maggie was dead, and it was many months before we spoke of her again. We'd breached a wall of hesitation in those few seconds. To my surprise, I soon found myself confiding to her about Salvador's and my little deceptions, our conspiracy of not reporting some of our study sites to Luis and Palma. She seemed genuinely tickled by the thought of it. She jumped up, still listening attentively, and brought us both a refill of brandy. Then she plopped herself down again beside me, perhaps just slightly more removed.

"That Salvador!" she said. "Shame on him for corrupting you. Eventually, you will discover that Salvador is kilotons smarter than Luis and Palma combined . . . probably smarter than Bucareli; or possibly Palma and Bucareli combined."

Then she began to tell me what she knew of Palma's horrendous program for killing all the snails in all the waterways of the island. Most alarming to me was the size of the program in men and matériel. One day at lunch, Gregorio had referred to some aspects of the program, but Gregorio's comments did not warn of anything of the magnitude that Emilia described.

I had pegged Gregorio to be about as tight-lipped a bureaucrat as any I'd known, and I mentioned this to Emilia.

"You must watch out for him," she said. "Very likely, he passes on to Palma every scrap of information that he gleans from any of the rest of us."

"What's his background?" I asked. "I mean, what's his education? What business was his father in?"

"He is the son of an importer. He attended the Liberal Arts Campus here in Aguilas and then went on to become a CPA."

"I wonder if he knows Charlie Bauer. Have you ever met Charlie Bauer?"

"Yes to both," she said. "And how did you come to know him?"

I described the plane trip and Charlie's curious comment about my needing help some day.

Emilia listened intently, but said nothing further about Gregorio or Charlie. In fact, she changed the subject abruptly—too abruptly it seemed to me. She brought the conversation around to Salvador's and my several field trips to Juncos.

"Could I go with you someday?" she asked. "I want to watch and see what you do when you are out in the field."

I suggested Wednesday of the following week. I explained that Salvador had another commitment that Wednesday. He would to be off to Comerio on the bus with two elderly women residents of Juncos who needed doctoring—apparently a sort of official mayoral function. Hence, I would have the Scout to myself.

I explained to Emilia that she might find the day kind of a drag since I was usually engrossed in my work and not much inclined to make small talk.

Just the same, Emilia jumped at the opportunity. "That would be perfect," she said, almost as though she was pleased I'd be distracted.

I felt obliged to warn her that I planned to do something a bit different on Wednesday. I planned to explore farther up into the headwaters of the *Perico* than Salvador and I had ever been before. There could be some personal danger to both of us. After all, there were supposed to be guerrilla forces, disloyal to the Bucareli leadership, lurking about up there in the *Espoleta*.

I explained further that Salvador had recently sketched a line on my topographic map that represented a potentially useful dirt and gravel road. He said he'd walked it many times, that it would be passable with the Scout. Instead of being directly associated with Juncos, however, the road began at the village of Valencia half-a-mile west of *Centrale Allende*. It extended north from Valencia up into the forest along the banks of a broad but shallow stream called the *Quebrada Segre*.

Halfway to its highest point, this primitive road branched, the right branch turning due east to intersect with tributaries of the *Perico* nearly a mile upstream from the village of Juncos.

Actually, the road led to an abandoned gold mine far up in the mountains above Juncos. I repeated that the adventure could be hazardous from several points of view, but that the Scout had 4-wheel drive and that would minimize the risk of getting stuck.

"That makes it even more perfect," she said.

Emilia and I set out Wednesday morning shortly after nine o'clock, as soon as I could gather my equipment together and check the Scout out of the motor pool. My plan required that we head for the Allende Bridge where all the sugar cane trucks must cross the *Ebro* with their harvest of cane for the factory. The bridge was a half-mile west of the factory. It was exactly 10 A.M. as we crossed it.

On the north side of the river we turned west. A half-mile west lay Valencia, a substantial grouping of stilted huts bordering the *Segre*. In the 1950s, Valencia was twice the size of Juncos. As at Juncos, the huts hugged the edge of the stream and were most heavily clustered close to where the *Segre* flows into the larger *Ebro*.

Salvador and I had collected snails at Valencia several times in the last several months. Many of these snails were infected and actively releasing cercariae. This was a prime place for transmission of the disease to humans and one that, for months, we carefully concealed both from Palma and Luis. In fact, Salvador and I had, on occasion, told little gray lies to Luis about the site when he inquired. I was determined to have my study sites. I considered this one essential.

Judging from my topographic map, I knew that the *Segre* occupies a huge watershed that reaches north into the *Espoleta* for a couple of miles, serving many hundreds of acres of upland valleys. This huge watershed offered endless opportunities for studying the biology of the snail and the dynamics of transmission of the disease to humans. Salvador and I planned to begin our study of the *Segre* the following week.

Heading north from Valencia up into the forest, we drove somewhat less than a mile along the dirt and gravel road that followed the main course of the *Segre.* Where the road branched, we turned east just as Salvador had sketched our route on my map. Working our way east and somewhat south for about half a mile, we were surprised to come upon a fork where a road branched off to the south and went steeply downhill. We parked the Scout here and walked downhill for about three hundred yards to discover that the branch-road led to a cliff just above *Centrale Allende*. Apparently, the road was once used to haul logs from the forest for the construction of the *centrale*. The timbers were lowered over the cliff by cables and winches more than a hundred feet down to the construction site. Concrete winch platforms still stood near the edge of the escarpment. The expensive winches had, of course, long since been removed.

We found that we could peer over the edge of Allende Cliff and see the awesome smokestack of the factory reaching up towards us like the raised trunk of a colossal mastodon from prehistoric time. From where we stood at the edge of the cliff, a person might be able to leap precisely into the gaping mouth of that huge smokestack with no more running start than a diver intending something as graceful as a swan dive.

From that fork, the main road continued east until it reached the abandoned gold mine high above Juncos. Salvador claimed that this mine was of great importance during the days of the Conquistadors. Although the vein had run out several hundred years ago, for some reason, possibly again to gain access to valuable timber, the road remained passable.

This rutted mountain road would prove a godsend for Salvador and me in the months that followed, enabling us to transport burdensome research equipment to the upper reaches of both the *Segre* and the *Perico*.

I must say I was thrilled with the prospects of the Valencia site. But I was also looking forward eagerly to what Emilia and I might find that day at the headwaters of the *Perico*. Salvador and I had discussed the enormous potential of both these upland locations many times. He had picked up immediately on my enthusiasm when I first mentioned the kind of studies I thought we would try to do. In fact, he was quick to say, "We no tell Luis. Okay?"

"*Absoluto!*" I had said. I was beginning to find words to use with Salvador that were not unlike their English equivalents—*invención*, *conexión*. The *-cion* words and their relatives proved worth their weight in Juncos gold. Salvador would fire them back at me. *Inspección?* expressed as a question meant *should we search for and determine the rate of infection of snails today. Religión, evolución*—we would discuss some pretty heady stuff on those long drives from Aguilas.

Mostly, one might say that we reflected on heady stuff without really much discourse. I'd say something about how the snail hosts had probably adapted over the years to a given environment.

He'd say, "*Evolución*," and cast me a knowing glance.

I'd say, "*Sí*," and we'd both slip into quiet meditation. After the interjection of a profound *ción* word like *evolu-*

ción, we might drive on for miles and miles until at last we stopped the Scout on a gravel wash to watch the sunlight dance across the eddies and riffles of our study stream as it spilled its crystalline waters into the muddy *Ebro*.

Beyond Allende Cliff, our rutted dirt and gravel road seemed almost a figment of one's imagination rather than a thoroughfare. Emilia and I ran into trouble when we tried to drive across a tributary, an upstream branch of the *Perico*, where loose sand had collected, probably from a recent storm. The rear tires of the Scout sank as though in quicksand down to the hubcaps. Gradually, I was able to work a number of branches and rotting log sections partially under all four tires and, in 4-wheel drive, with Emilia at the wheel and me pushing, we managed to get on with our journey. However, it was after three o'clock in the afternoon when we reached the abandoned gold mine and parked in the subdued light of typically dense tropical rain forest.

That day became one of the most exciting days of my life. Dipping for snails as we followed the *Perico* upstream through the forest, we found them abundant in all stages of growth.

Perhaps we dawdled a bit along the way, because it was four o'clock when we reached a broad, nearly level expanse of just over half an acre, approximately a hundred and fifty feet on a side, where the uppermost waters of the *Perico* seeped from the base of a huge wall of rock and collected in the hoof prints of horses and cattle.

In each hoof print we found snails of all sizes along with abundant gelatinous egg masses. The egg masses were attached to twigs below the surface of the water or glued to the underside of leaves floating on the water. In short, we stood in the midst of a snail breeding ground of enormous importance.

I had speculated on the existence of such sites in other countries. However, I had never before actually seen one. Undoubtedly, this protected habitat of tiny breeding chambers, these hoof prints, explained vividly how snail repopulation downstream could occur repeatedly and so quickly after every storm.

In the weeks that followed, Salvador and I were to prove this quiet habitat to be exactly that. He and I would spend hundreds of hours amongst those hoof prints marking snails' shells with brightly colored, fast-drying lacquer paints, and many hundreds of additional hours dipping for snails downstream and finding our painted snails in practically every protected pool all the way down to the confluence with the *Rio Ebro*. This was a discovery of incalculable interest.

This seepage area beneath that giant wall of rock so high up into the *Espoleta* seemed an odd spot to find livestock, especially cattle. Horses, yes, perhaps, but cattle raising was essentially restricted to the lower coastal plains. I was intrigued almost as much with that aspect of our discovery as with the presence of breeding snails. "I don't get it," I said. "They must be strays."

"Quite some distance for cattle to stray," Emilia said. "The nearest herd I know of is close to Madoz, and Madoz is maybe six kilometers west of here on the coast and at sea level. We must be well over four hundred meters elevation."

"Close to five," I suggested.

We counted contour lines on my topographic map. We were almost at six hundred meters, over eighteen hundred feet above sea level. We hadn't walked but a short distance from where we parked the Scout beside the entrance to the gold mine. The section of road between Allende Cliff and the gold mine must have been deceivingly steep.

Twilight comes early to the Caribbean, and with the twilight comes a change in mood. One senses one's own relaxation as the tensions of the day begin to wind down. This initial relief from the stress of the day is followed by a heightening of consciousness. Sounds seem amplified as the light fades. The call of the nightjar at dusk, and his mate's reply, a duet that would hardly be noticed if it occurred in the heat of the day, comes towards evening to totally capture a listener's attention.

In our open, boggy meadow we still had plenty of light; yet, in my excitement over finding such a huge population of breeding snails, we had tarried longer than was wise. Salvador and I had often worked this late into the afternoon, but never at this elevation, with miles of dirt and gravel forest road between us and the nearest blacktop.

Just as we decided to head back to the Scout, we were startled by a chilling, muffled, metallic sound. It took me a moment to place it. Someone close by had chambered a round in a bolt-action weapon.

Two men dressed in olive-drab fatigues and armed with what looked like cast-off WWII infantry carbines stood blocking our path back to the Scout. I glanced at Emilia. She'd seen them before I had. Her body had suddenly pressed against me. For a moment, I held my breath. She took my hand and laced her fingers through mine.

"Marcos Díaz!" she whispered.

My eyes questioned hers. She squeezed my hand, again, saying, "Marcos Díaz!" emphasizing the surname as though certainly I would comprehend its importance.

"Which one?" I asked, remembering at last this name from news releases several years ago.

"On the left."

"You know him?" It was a dumb comment. Clearly, she knew him. She was alarmed, but oddly, didn't seem the least bit frightened.

I took a step toward the two men. She tried to restrain me, but I shook my hand free and took another step or two. They hadn't advanced. Nor had they bothered to raise their rifles. I turned, intending to tell Emilia to stay put.

As I turned, I noticed that behind us, at the northwest edge of the meadow, about a dozen men dressed in army fatigues had taken up positions against the face of the rock wall. They were standing at ease, rifle butts resting on the damp ground. As I looked, one lit a cigarette. Clearly, they didn't expect us to charge them with dip-nets. But how or when they had gotten there, I don't know. They simply materialized. In any case, escape by that route was out of the question.

I couldn't leave Emilia standing like a startled fawn near the edge of the clearing. I returned to her and took her hand again. "Let's assume," I said, "that if they intended us any harm they'd have already shot us or rushed us or whatever they do when they catch somebody up here."

I now began to recall that this Marcos Díaz fellow was always portrayed by the American press as more of an intellectual and visionary than a rebel.

Our press liked him; our government didn't.

I'd read brief accounts of him. Curiously, he held a doctorate in tropical medicine from none other than Tulane, possibly the most prestigious place in the United States—if not the world—to study tropical medicine.

In addition, he had a law degree from someplace in California. I'd always assumed that he was dead; probably killed years ago in a clash with government troops. As he was alive, it was a given that I would encounter him eventually. Just my bad luck to come face to face with him on the very day I chose to invite Emilia to accompany me, and on a day when Salvador was not along to provide the measure of sage advice necessary to get through the introductions safely.

Emilia was shivering. "I'm just nervous from being so easily surprised," she said. "There will be no reason for them to harm us as long as *you* keep your wits about you and behave."

"Unless, from their point of view, knowing their whereabouts up here puts us in danger."

"Bucareli knows they are here. However, Bucareli does not know their strength, how many are here or what ordinance they have. Hence, I agree, it is better that we, especially you, do not see more than we have already."

"Then we'd best head home." I was surprised that Emilia accepted so easily that they were here.

"Lead on," she said, once again weaving her delicate fingers between mine.

Marcos Díaz seemed to be enjoying our plight as we approached. I remember him at that moment as extremely alert and smiling, as though looking forward to the encounter. He was a small man, a head shorter than I, stocky, muscular, probably somewhere around one-hundred-and-sixty pounds. He appeared close to my age, perhaps a few years older, maybe in his late thirties, clean and clean-shaven.

His army fatigues made him seem no different from those behind us against the face of the rock wall, or, for that matter, than Salvador on any ordinary day of fieldwork. Except that Salvador was eighty, and the side pockets of his fatigues bulged with bottles of rubbing alcohol for our hands and arms rather than grenades and clips of ammunition.

We drew to within fifteen feet of him before he spoke. "Doctor Livingstone, I presume?"

"Perhaps I'm the one who should be saying that to you," I told him. He'd broken the ice with passive humor, albeit perhaps a bit sarcastic. I was grateful to him for sparing our lives to that point at least.

Looking back on that encounter now from a span of over forty-five years, I recall that after that first exchange my composure completely returned. I should point out that Marcos's special interest at Tulane was malaria. He and Emilia had that in common. He'd earned his doctorate in

1948, returned briefly to Tavira, then left abruptly for California where he studied political science and law. About 1951 he returned to Tavira and worked vigorously to try to persuade the legislature to impeach incumbent leader Juan Bucareli.

Bucareli's title was that of president, but he was clearly a dictator. He had been in office since the '30s and apparently had no intention of giving up the reins to a pipsqueak dreamer who had spent essentially all of his adult life in the States.

Then, in 1953, Marcos mysteriously disappeared. The official word was that he had gone elsewhere to seek his fortune—possibly Central or South America. Yet, as I've said, I simply assumed that Bucareli had succeeded in having him killed.

In Aguilas, the existence of guerrillas in the *Espoleta* was largely considered a myth. Apparently, it was only among high officials of the government and among the rural folk such as Salvador, living along the base of the *Espoleta*, that their presence had credibility.

"And if it isn't little Madame Curie herself," Marcos said. "What a thrill to have this unexpected visit from you!" Oddly, he winked at her.

"Get down off your high horse, Marcos," Emilia told him. "Say quickly what you have to say. Doctor Livingstone has to get back to Aguilas before the motor pool closes, and we are running late."

"I could accuse you and *el doctor* of trespassing and have you both put in our bamboo jail for a few days. How would that suit you, Emilia?"

"Some other time!"

Somehow or other, Marcos knew Emilia, and vice versa—perhaps from early school days. Obviously, he knew something about her present employment. I sensed they were speaking in English mostly for my benefit. However, what surprised me most were Emilia's aggressive responses. She was countering him even more assertively than I'd seen her deal with Palma on so many occasions over the past few months.

I'd have expected that a man like Palma might fire an employee as consistently contrary and combative as Emilia. And it didn't seem as though Marcos Díaz, of all people, needed to put up with her for an instant.

She had guts, I decided. There was no doubt about that. Even here in the camp of the enemy, she said just about whatever came into her head. Yet, she'd selectively warned *me* about keeping *my* wits. Just then, I would have preferred that she be a bit more assuaging.

The next thing he said to her was, "I will allow you to pass if you promise to do me one favor."

"Don't try to bribe me! I prefer to hear you beg. I might surprise you."

"Okay then, I beg." Hand to the waist, he bowed deeply. "Tell the honorable *el señor* jackass Palma that to squirt his toxic chemicals around anywhere in the *Espoleta* is going to make me very cross with him."

She looked straight at him with that same wooden stare that I'd watched her use on Palma. "Marcos, I have a surprise for you. Palma means business. We no longer have the slack to convince him otherwise. Harvey, here, can confirm that. I have tried on several occasions. Harvey tried. We were both shot down.

"Nevertheless, I will pass it along, but perhaps not as bluntly as you wish. I will explain to him that *if you exist* you probably will not stand by and let him spray. I am not supposed to know you exist, or so you keep telling me!"

"It has to be stronger than that *this time*, Emilia."

What caught my attention were the words: *this time*.

"It is time to stop playing games, Emilia," he said. "I am asking you to tell him about this specific encounter in full detail."

"But, Marcos—"

"You saw me. I'm here. I'm standing here telling you to tell Palma to back off. We are not talking revolution here. We are talking *do not spray snails with SCP.* If he complies, then we ask nothing more. Salvador tells me that he is confident that Harvey, here, can formulate an effective plan for control if he is given time to complete even a reasonable study. But, in the meantime, Palma must be convinced that inconceivable damage will be done to the ecology of the *Espoleta* by this crazy massive treatment with chemicals. If he hasn't the brains to give up the idea then we will have to . . . we will have to take appropriate action at the appropriate time." He grinned his compelling grin and added, "That's a phrase I learned in first-year law school. I love it!"

"That is nice, Marcos. Very funny. Good for you," Emilia said.

He raised his rifle and fired a round into the air. Promptly, the men near the rock wall filed off into the woods. "I am serious, Emilia. Either he quits this insane scheme or he's going to accidentally get himself killed. I will personally appear one day in Aguilas and ring the bastard's fat neck!"

Emilia was obviously quite at ease with him. "*Sí, señor,*" she said, miming a compliant servant who sought her master's sanction.

I was surprised to learn that Marcos knew Salvador and had recently spoken with him. And the most important thing about that revelation was that Marcos had high regard for advice he received from Salvador.

So that was it! Juan Bucareli, with his retinue of bodyguards and his army, might be reasonably content to leave the guerrillas alone for the present, but Harlan Palma was not safe from the lengthening arm of Marcos Díaz. Palma could not harm Emilia without retribution from Marcos, and presumably Palma already knew that.

As I watched the two of them, I began to realize that somehow they must be related. At least their friendship went way back.

Then, for some odd reason, I couldn't help myself and said, "Doctor, please tell me why, when your people steal a man's wallet, you replace his small denomination bills with new hundreds." Immediately, I felt like a fool. Here we were talking shop with a guerrilla about snails, assassination, and revolution, a fantastically revealing experience, and I had to come up with an asinine question like that. I looked at him rather sheepishly.

He grinned. "Pinned that on me, did you?" Then he said, "That is one we will save for our next conference. Emilia is right. You are running late. Pacheco here will accompany you as far as the *Segre* . . . Is that Salvador's usual Scout you are driving?"

"Yes."

"Then it has 4-wheel drive. You should be okay. However, Pacheco will go along to push just in case you get stuck a second time."

I looked at him carefully. So he'd had us under surveillance most of the day. And he wanted me to know that.

I thanked him for his concern that we get safely to Valencia, and I moved on past him to lead the way. We were *definitely* running late. The motor pool closed at 8 P.M. Of course, I could always claim that we encountered engine trouble or ran out of gas.

On an impulse, I turned. I did so just in time to see Emilia hug Marcos quickly.

His eyes met mine. He said, "Harvey, thank you for bringing her today. I hope I did not frighten you too badly. We have much to talk about, you and I."

Apparently, we did. I was curious to know how the two of them had arranged this supposedly spontaneous encounter.

I wasn't destined to learn that right away.

Dangerous Waters

During my brief nine days in Puerto Rico with Sam, I watched Sam construct an ingenious filtering device for measuring the number of cercariae in samples of water collected from rivers and streams. He invented it piece-by-piece, devoting after-work hours and one entire weekend to prowling the aisles of hardware and kitchen-appliance stores in contemplation of unorthodox uses for the stuff he saw there. Gradually, he converted an ordinary household pressure cooker into a pressure filter by drilling a thousand holes in the bottom and substituting a garden hose connection for the steam valve in the top. Basically, the device forced a measured quantity of water through carefully selected filter paper. Then, the operator had only to heat-stain the filter paper with a stain called ninhydrin that colors proteins and not much else. He constructed two of these devices in less than a week.

Stained cercariae, trapped by the filter paper, appeared purple against the white background and could be quickly counted using a dissecting microscope at a magnification even as low as twenty times. Of course, it was not possible to say that all of the cercariae trapped on the paper were one or another of the human species of schistosome. However, in practiced hands, the importance of the concept could not be underestimated.

Before boarding the plane for my flight from Puerto Rico to Tavira the previous June, Sam surprised me with the gift of one of these contraptions. As I promised in my letter to him, written during the flight to Aguilas, I would surely put the device, which he called a *cercariometer*, to good use. At first, Salvador and I referred to it as our *olla de presión*, but we eventually simplified that to just *the filter*.

Salvador and I tested the filter several times at Juncos both before and after Luis sprayed with SCP. We also used it at other sites on numerous occasions. In fact it became our primary tool for locating transmission sites. We learned that most of these sites produced maybe a dozen cercariae per gallon. Valencia was the exception.

We first sampled the *Segre* at Valencia during a thunderstorm. The rain constantly soaked our hands. Because of this, it was difficult to keep track of when we also accidentally got our hands wet with water from the stream. For Salvador, growing up in Juncos with constant exposure to infection, this did not pose the danger that it did for me. People frequently exposed to just a few cercariae at a time over many years develop considerable immunity. We know that now. We suspected it back then.

Routinely, we both applied isopropyl alcohol to our hands when we accidentally got them wet with stream water. Worldwide, in those days, most schisto workers did this. Any exposure was dangerous back then. There simply were no satisfactory drugs for treating the disease, and, as with some of the chemotherapy drugs of today, treatment could become very unpleasant. Fortunately, they have some excellent drugs for schisto today.

Back then, many of us believed that, if untreated, an initial dose of as few as two hundred cercariae, maturing into adult worms in the victim's abdomen, could kill a newcomer to the disease. I didn't know how accurate that guess might be, but I was reluctant to play the role of guinea pig.

Salvador and I decided that we should collect our water samples for the filter from the middle of the stream. In a broad stream such as the *Segre*, this meant wading out over slippery rocks to a point about fifteen feet from shore, poking the intake hose down in the water, and keeping it submerged for several minutes while one's partner worked the hand pump back on dry land.

Wearing hip boots, I struck out for the middle of the *Segre*, rain splashing about me as I stepped gingerly over the moss-covered stones.

I had been out there for about five minutes when Salvador encountered some trouble with the filter. I went ashore to help, then back out. However, on the way back out I slipped, caught myself, and shipped perhaps a half-gallon of water over the top of my left boot. The water soaked my pant leg and socks. I ignored it. After all, I figured, perhaps less than a dozen cercariae might be involved, and maybe all of them would get stuck in the weave of my thin trousers and fail to reach my skin.

To heat-stain the wet filter paper when working in the field, we'd lift the paper circle out of the filter and lay it on a twelve-inch pizza pan in a little pool of the stain. Then, with heat protective gloves, we'd hold the pan by its edge over a can of sand soaked with burning naphtha, an old army trick for heating C-rations. When the paper had steamed bone dry, the staining process was complete.

The Valencia count? . . . We had recovered one-hundred-and-thirty-two cercariae per gallon of stream water—a lethal dose in every gallon and a half. I was in big trouble! The moment the itching and rash began the length of my left leg I knew it was too late for the isopropyl alcohol to do any good.

How the weeks dragged as I waited to discover the severity of my infection. Over subsequent weeks, eggs appeared in my stools in ever increasing numbers. Fever seemed a constant companion, and bouts of diarrhea tethered me to the toilets of Tavira so tightly that I dared not climb out of the Scout without first spotting a restroom, or in the field, an outhouse.

I wondered if my abdomen would expand like a watermelon as it does in the rural children living along the infected streams. Doctor Palma's heartening advice (which he swore to be impartial) was to let it go untreated. "Nothing to it, Harvey," he said. "You should be good as new in a dozen years."

Paranoia gripped me in my worst moments of abdominal agony as I imagined my recall so close on the heels of Ota Homma. Was Palma mean-minded enough to plot my recall in such a spineless way, knowing how painfully I'd die? The prognosis did not look good. Nevertheless, I took his advice and chose not to undergo treatment.

By some miracle, my infection turned out to be a light one. It did resolve itself in a dozen years just as Palma had predicted, God rest his soul. It goes to prove that even a scoundrel can't free himself of some inherent good.

The adult schistosome worms do not multiply in humans. The severity of an infection depends solely on how many cercariae penetrate the skin, make their way to the blood vessels surrounding the intestine, and mature into egg-laying females. Apparently, it's the thousands upon thousands of spiny eggs that do most of the damage as they work their way like tiny barbed daggers through the walls of the blood vessels and into the intestine.

That fantastically high cercarial count at Valencia tempted us to want to know how the number of cercariae in the water might differ at different hours of the day and night. Testing every half hour for twenty-four hours might produce some interesting results. Salvador was excited over the prospect. All we needed was clearance from Palma to keep the Scout out of the motor pool overnight. We swore ourselves to secrecy, adopted a code name for Valencia, removed all maps and notes from the Scout each evening upon our return from the field, and made certain each morning that we were not followed as we set out. The *Segre* had become our diamond in the rough.

Pidal's Appropriation

I had now been working on the island of Tavira for six months. In mid-December on a Monday morning, Harlan Palma called a general meeting of the Department of Health in the auditorium on the first floor. I was not forewarned. Luckily, I had planned to look some things up in the Department library that day. I got wind of the meeting when the librarian closed up shop to attend.

Since Palma had not invited me to be present on stage along with Luis, Emilia, and Gregorio, I found a seat near the back of the auditorium. As the employees gathered, Palma waited in silence at the podium. Staff members were checking attendance at the door. Every few minutes, Palma would pace the stage once or twice and then return to the podium.

Finally, the signal came that essentially everyone was present. Palma called the meeting to order. Loosely translated, he said, "Ladies and gentlemen, today we embark on perhaps the most exciting task in the history of our Department. *El señor* Felipe Pidal has agreed to introduce a bill in the Senate that will budget twelve million pesos for the eradication of the snail, *Australorbis glabratus*, from

Tavira's rivers and streams." The exchange rate at the time was two pesos to the dollar.

Applause broke out. Whether spontaneous or initiated by carefully planted supporters, the applause spread throughout the room. I couldn't believe the response. Had any of them even considered the downside of such a massive project?

There was no question about it, Palma had charisma, and his power base within the government was just about to take a giant step forward.

Our leader continued, "This funding will make possible enormous changes in the Department. We are planning to purchase fifty specialized field vehicles and the very latest in high-pressure spray equipment. We will hire over two hundred new employees. In addition, of course, and just as a beginning, we will purchase half a ton of the chemical used to kill the snails. And, of course, we require hundreds of additional dip-nets, waders, gloves, and uniforms."

Palma's program was ten times the size I had considered likely. The hints I'd had from Emilia and Gregorio were nowhere near that high. Half a ton of SCP correctly diluted! That was probably enough to poison the Yangtze River all the way to Burma. The man was insane! They might get several years use out of the trucks and spray tanks, but they'd be embarking on a program they'd have to repeat not only every year but more likely after every modest rainstorm.

There were less than half-a-dozen questions from the floor. Only two touched on environmental issues. A woman asked if the chemical would make the water in the streams poisonous to drink. A man asked if the chemical would injure young stands of sugar cane as the *Copper sulfate* had done in the past. Palma made light of the first, skillfully avoiding the word *cancer* as he spoke. The second question, he dealt with in more detail, pointing out that SCP seems to be more of an animal poison than a plant poison. Then he summed up the discussion by pointing out that his *lieutenants* were on top of all of these questions and would be happy to provide detailed information to those few who might be interested. Finally, he reminded them that it was essential that everyone work together as a team.

At the end of the general meeting, Palma called a private meeting in his office for just himself, Luis, Gregorio, Emilia, and me. Since I was not made aware of the general meeting, I'm sure I was invited to the private meeting primarily so that he could lambaste me again regarding my supposed role in the project, that of finding sites and doing post-treatment sampling. No doubt, he intended to occupy every moment of my tour of duty on Tavira with these two monotonous tasks. No doubt, he would see to it that I hadn't an instant to spare or a scrap of energy left for basic research.

My guess proved correct. He stressed my role several times. "And Doctor Shoals will be our birddog, pointing out transmission sites and tracking our successes. We could not undertake this complex campaign without him."

Did the others agree with this monstrous plan? If, during the planning stages, he had sought the expertise of his senior staff, I might at least have found it possible to trust his motivation even if not his judgment. But he had not consulted with his senior staff. The thing was done completely without input from Luis, Emilia, or Gregorio.

One thing was certain: with such an enormous boost in personnel and equipment, he would control the largest department of the government. More than that, if he were to use the opportunity to full advantage—perhaps to tramp around in the villages seeking grassroots support—he could generate a bountiful number of votes.

Elections were just over a year away. It seemed likely that he had been planning for some time to contest Bucareli for the presidency in January of 1960, and that this new program was intended as a stepping-stone in that direction.

I was depressed before the private meeting began. I grew more depressed as the meeting continued. I could hardly bring myself to say what I felt I had to say. Finally, for perhaps the fifth or sixth time, I stressed that killing the snails could only be considered a temporary measure. They would return in force.

"Thank you, Doctor," Palma said, his anger obvious in the intonation as he continued. "Shoals, I think we have had a prolific and sufficient accounting of that point of view. Partially proven presumptions add little to a discussion. I hope we will discover that you can be a team player, even if you do not agree on all the particulars."

"Doctor Palma," Emilia began, "much of the work of those spray teams is going to have to be done in the valleys of the *Espoleta*."

"Your point?"

"Is it possible that there could be guerrilla elements in those valleys who would not take kindly to the concept of poisoning the waters of a hundred streams and their tributaries."

Palma belittled her. "Oh come now, Emilia. We must not get into the habit of parroting Harvey by inferring that we will be *poisoning* these waterways. At the dilution we're using, even your tender skin would remain as lovely as ever.

"And another thing, Emilia, there is no need to be so coy. We all know the crazy bastard is up there." He stopped to concentrate on scraping the bowl of his pipe with a pocketknife, dumping the fragments of charred tobacco in the ashtray on the coffee table in front of him. "You would not be aware of it, Emilia, but President Bucareli has already initiated plans that will terminate any possible intervention by the guerrillas. I am speaking of *significant* plans. The president intends to annihilate Marcos Díaz and his criminal cronies step-by-step, both those in the *Espoleta* and also his confederates here in the city. The estimated wrap-up date for that operation is set to coincide with the elections."

Emilia looked directly at him but said nothing in response.

Obviously, he was quite pleased with himself, and had no doubts that Pidal's legislation would pass. Then he came up with a shocker, at least for me.

"I have also just learned from President Bucareli that, starting immediately, every time Luis ventures out to spray a stream, and every day Harvey and Salvador take to the field in the Scout, they will be protected at their work site by a platoon of well-armed and well-trained infantry. I am to report to division headquarters in Comerio a full twenty-four hours in advance so that these platoons can be dispatched in time to secure the perimeter of the work site. What do you think of that?" He looked carefully at each of us in turn.

"What that means," he added, "is that I need to know your schedules for every day of the week a full two days in advance." As he spoke he passed Luis and me packets of forms on which to schedule our field trips. "Include exactly where you are going, when you will arrive at your destination, who will be with you, and how long you estimate your work will take."

"I can't believe this," I said. "I never know in advance exactly where I'm going to be working! Each field trip depends on a lot of other circumstances and often on the results gleaned the previous day. That's an absurd request!"

"Like it or not, that's how it's going to be," Palma said. "Maybe this is the point at which you need to make some tough decisions. We would be severely handicapped, but I'm sure we can manage without you."

I ignored his implication and returned to the basic point of dissention, that SCP would destroy all animal life in the rivers and streams. Hundreds of thousands of fish would be killed, just to mention one factor. "Your rural folk depend on these fish as a regular part of their diet. I've also seen them catching crayfish and especially the river crab, the *siwik* I think they call it. Furthermore, you have numerous bird species that fish the streams and estuaries. And that includes your priceless mangrove habitats, most of which receive freshwater from one or another of your rivers. What a tragedy it would be if SCP applied to the rivers got into the mangroves! You are proposing a program that—"

"One of the problems I have with visiting scientists, especially you PDS people," Palma was developing a nasty habit of drowning me out in mid-sentence with a shrill raised voice, "is that they arrive with a big chip on each shoulder. If I complain about their officiousness they go back to the hotel to get a bigger set of chips, big as the coasters at the bar at the Mar Chiquita where they hang out most of the night before dragging in here about time for mid-morning coffee. Apparently, they are born with an endless bundle of objections to anything they haven't themselves conceived."

That little speech went all over me. I hadn't set foot in the bar at the Mar Chiquita, and I felt I'd been carrying my share of the workload at least as well as Luis or Gregorio and certainly better than the allegedly obnoxious Ota Homma. "I don't mean to be officious," I said. "It's just that on an island as small as Tavira, when you tamper with one aspect of the environment you stand the chance of upsetting other factors that may be especially important to the quality of life. This is a powerful chemical. Biologists are stepping back from using it almost everywhere throughout the world. I'm shocked and saddened that you would even consider using it here."

"Shoals, we have been over and over this ad nauseam!" He picked up a book and slammed it down on the desk. "Damn you academic pinheads! Either you get smart, Shoals, and start cooperating or I will have you shipped back to Geneva on a container ship, preferably in a small container of your own."

Luis and Gregorio were silent throughout this exchange, but I knew Luis felt at least as intimidated as I. As an accountant, Gregorio could work effectively within any branch of the government. He hadn't been with the Department of Health long. Briefly, I wondered if Bucareli might have purposely posted Gregorio to the Department of Health, perhaps with orders to keep a close eye on Palma's activities. I'd do that, I thought to myself, if I were the autocratic leader of a country and discovered I had a loose cannon rolling about in my most important department.

The session ended. Palma had been rough on Emilia several times during the meeting, yet, I noticed as the meeting broke up that he went out of his way to be pleasant to her. I wondered how long it would take her to reach Marcos with the news of Bucareli's alleged decision to move against the guerrillas, or to inform him of the platoons of infantry that would be dogging Luis and me in the field. I wondered how many men there were in a Taviran platoon, how they would be armed, and how that might sit with the locals.

It would be several weeks before I saw much of Emilia as I felt it crucial that Salvador and I push ahead with the cercarial studies immediately.

Incidentally, I forgot to mention another crucial decision that came out of that meeting. Before the announcement about the platoon of infantry that would accompany our fieldwork, I asked Palma directly if Salvador and I could sometimes keep the Scout out of the motor pool overnight. I made the excuse that we needed to get an early start if we were to reach certain of the more remote streams of the *Espoleta*. His answer was an instant and emphatic *no*.

AROUND THE CLOCK

Salvador and I wasted no time getting to the hourly studies that would reveal when cercariae were most abundant in the water. He agreed to meet me at *Centrale Allende* about seven thirty on Wednesday morning. Because we were forbidden to keep the Scout overnight, I leased a Volkswagen Beetle from a garage around the corner from the hotel. It was a poor choice for our gear. The snail dippers wouldn't fit in the bonnet, so they occupied the back seat with the handles extending out the front window on Salvador's side.

Salvador walked from Juncos, joining a group of sugar cane workers on their way to the *centrale*. I drove the Volkswagen across the *Ebro* at the Allende Bridge, picked him up at the factory gate, and then the two of us rode to Valencia.

We arrived at Valencia with about ten minutes to spare for sorting out our gear before drawing the eight o'clock sample. Salvador readied the pump and hose. I set up the dissecting microscope on one side of our small field table while, across from me, Salvador got the pizza pan and naphtha burner ready so that I could do the staining quickly and then move right around to the microscope to make the count. I figured I could easily complete each count before time to draw the next sample.

The eight o'clock, half past eight, and nine o'clock samples came in completely negative. I thought I had one cercaria on the nine o'clock sample, but if it were a cercaria, its forked tail had broken away.

There were a few cercariae in the 9:30 sample. Then the real excitement began. By noon we were getting counts of over one hundred cercariae per gallon. Counts at these levels continued until three o'clock at which time we began to notice a decline.

By 5:30 P.M., cercariae were mostly gone from the samples. We were thrilled with the results. We hadn't expected nearly so much variation. But where had the cercariae gone?

In our excitement, the afternoon passed quickly, and cane workers began arriving home from the fields shortly after we drew the 5:30 sample. They were a talkative lot, and seemed in high spirits, as though the day had gone well and the work had tired them little. All were muscular and trim. Each carried a carefully cleaned and razor-sharp machete, the primary tool of their trade. They'd been thinning fields of young cane and repairing irrigation channels between the rows.

I soon experienced firsthand their deep curiosity regarding schisto. I doubt they'd ever seen an *americano* streamside, hovering over a dissecting microscope, and taking turns wading out into the *Segre* to hold the end of the intake hose midstream.

After they got the picture of what we were doing, they had to see everything. We showed them the noon sample with its multitude of cercariae glistening blue against the white, unstained background of the filter paper. In their gracious, rural way, they looked and more or less pretended to see. Some, no doubt, saw them, but getting used to using a dissecting scope takes a bit of practice.

The old snail-in-the-beaker routine worked better for them. "*Dios mío!*" they'd exclaim, peering into a water glass alive with a thousand shimmering cercariae.

Those who could manage the dissecting scope couldn't leave it. "*Qué es esto?*" "*Qué es eso?*" we'd hear as they squinted usually through just one eyepiece. "*Dónde, Dónde?*" another would crowd in. I was practically in tears from the emotion of watching their enthusiasm. What a snap it would be to educate them once we'd assembled our facts.

Salvador had obtained the rank of full professor in their eyes even before the sun set. I think no one left our side until darkness enveloped our little campus. They'd learned the fun of holding the cercariae-filled water glass up to the light from the fast fading sunset in the west—a truly remarkable 3D effect of motion and refracted color. Then, as they left, there were many sincere expressions of "*Gracias!*" and "*Gracias por su paciencia.*"

A few of the men and some of their wives came back to watch us after their evening meal. The women asked a host of questions, and I had never seen Salvador so talkative or so much in command of his audience. He was superb, and he appeared to love every minute of it. Of course, he was the mayor of the neighboring village. They all knew it. But as I look back in time to that most wonderful of moments in my entire career, I realize that he held a trump card vastly more important than that of being a mayor of Juncos. He was the companion of the *loco gringo* who found the banks of the *Segre* more to his liking than the nightclubs and casinos of Aguilas.

By the light of our gas lantern, we could show the wives the midday filter papers, and we still had the midday, water-filled jars with their shimmering larvae that rose and fell in a rhythm of patient and treacherous anticipation.

They could watch and understand our filtration procedure; and, most important, they observed firsthand that there were no cercariae in those evening samples.

I could follow some of what this new clutch of visitors had to say. One aggressive young mother was far more outspoken than the others. She spoke in English, probably so that she could watch my immediate reaction to her words. "All the time they tell us 'stay out of water.' Make children stay out of water. How you make children stay out of water?"

Salvador answered her question by adapting what we were just now learning to her situation. Namely, that if our data were correct, the water was rather safe most hours of the day. The bad time would be in the heat of the day.

Biologists already knew that cercariae were killed by only a trace of chlorine in water. I brought in this idea and Salvador translated it. No doubt rural women could be taught to add a few drops of ordinary bleach to water drawn from the stream if they really had to use water collected during the midday hours. In seconds, just a few drops of bleach per gallon would render the water safe. This translated into just pennies per year, and bleach was on the shelf of every grocery store, rural as well as in the cities. No doubt they even carried it in the store at the *centrale*.

If the predictable presence of cercariae that we observed that day turned out to be a universal rule, then water could be drawn during safe hours into streamside retainers for use during the heat of the day. Certainly there were dozens of directions to take our new information if it really did prove to be true.

"Why Health Department no tell us about bleach?" the same woman asked. "They order us around. Stay out of water. Why no tell us something we *can* do? Why all time tell us what *not* to do?"

That, to be sure, was the sixty-four dollar question. It has been my observation that in young nations that are just starting on the road to industrialization, many lower-echelon health employees, working their hard-won new jobs, are reluctant to curb the urge to wield authority.

The gathering thinned out before 10 P.M. and eventually darkness found us alone with a long night's stand yet to go.

Occasionally, from one of the stilted huts, we'd hear a child cry out, a parent speak. There was the metallic ping of a saucepan as someone tried to capture the last heat from charcoal embers. Then a lovely voice—perhaps a lullaby. And finally, almost as an anthem to mark the end of day, a woman sang a portion of my favorite solo from *La Boheme* with a beauty I had never ever heard before, and perhaps because of that magical setting, with a beauty I don't expect that I shall ever hear again.

Towards midnight a pair of nightjars began to arrange a rendezvous, their rasping calls scarcely minutes apart—the proposal from the east bank; affirmation from the west.

In the wee hours, collecting samples soon fell into a monotonous routine. We lit our pressurized gas lantern each half hour to obtain enough light for the dissecting scope. A clear sky and partly full moon provided all the light we needed for our other tasks. All through the remainder of the night, no cercariae appeared on the papers. Not one!

As we rested between samples, sometimes even napping—hard gravel beneath our backs—we speculated on what had happened to the cercarial population. If cercariae can live in a glass of water for many hours, why had they disappeared so suddenly and completely from the stream?

Salvador posed the obvious. "Sun makes them come out of snails. Sun goes away; cercariae go away."

"Yes, but they would still be in the water *around* the snails," I said.

"They go downstream into *Rio Ebro*."

"But it stands to reason that many would remain in the submerged vegetation *near* the snails along the edge of the stream where there is practically no current or where an occasional eddy might cause them to remain more or less indefinitely in place."

Reluctantly, considering how tired we were, we decided to find out. For several hours, we took our usual center-stream sample and also a composite second sample from points chosen at random along the edge of the stream. Sample after sample came up negative.

At precisely two o'clock in the morning, as I selected my footholds gingerly among the submerged stones and worked my way to the center of the stream, I sensed the sound of a footstep somewhere near the Volkswagen. *Sensed* is accurate. I thought I'd heard the almost imperceptible crunch of a heavy boot on smooth, round gravel. Salvador must have heard it, too. His back was to me. He was facing the Volkswagen.

A familiar voice said, "Aha! Doctor Livingstone. *Bueno!* I expected I'd find you intent on some nefarious sporting venture around here somewhere. Don't they have a pool back at the hotel?"

"Greetings, Marcos. You're just in time to cash in on what we've learned," I said, as I held the hose in the water while Salvador pumped the sample. "However," I added, "if you plan again to try to shoot me, I beg you to wait till morning. What we are coming up with here is absolutely fantastic!"

"I find it hard to comprehend devotion to duty in a *gringo* sufficient to cause him to work through a long hot night even in as pleasant a setting as Valencia. I have been watching you with binoculars from the ridge practically all afternoon. Curiosity got the best of me when you failed to leave. What is so critical that you can't let it wait until morning?"

"Marcos, we are in the process of discovering something completely unexplainable."

"Well then, my apologies for interrupting. I mostly wanted to see if you had about you a platoon of soldiers. I see you don't. That is, unless they are off napping somewhere in the bushes."

"So you've been expecting that sort of thing?" I said.

"Napping? No indeed."

"Infantry."

"Yes. I got the word. Our mutual friend."

I assumed he meant Emilia, but how did Emilia contact him? "Very likely we'd have had the infantry with us, but Herr Palma doesn't know we're out, so to speak."

That seemed to delight him and he had a good laugh. "I noticed you didn't bring the Scout," he said.

"Palma won't let it out of the motor pool overnight."

"What a pity! I'd hoped perhaps you might occasionally agree to bring us a box of ammo. Traveling at night, it would be so much safer. You could anyway, you know. I can put you in touch with a source. But the size box I have in mind would not fit in your Beetle."

I ignored that suggestion. "How does 'our mutual friend' contact you? Radio?"

"Please, Harvey! I want you to relay a message. Please tell her to always use *the alternative message route* from now on. The powers that be are beginning to get nasty. I don't like the looks of things."

"*The alternative message route,* those exact words? "

"Yes. Those are the operative words."

"I'll mention it. Thanks for caring." I said.

"Are you aware of the insurmountable damage Palma will do if he treats these streams with his infernal chemical?" Marcos asked. "He absolutely must be stopped. It is politics that drives him. He's not stupid enough to fail to understand what a disaster SCP is going to cause."

"I came to the same conclusion after a meeting we had the other day. I mean, as to how it's politics that's driving him. But I can't stop him. He's developed a keen dislike for me. In fact, I'm afraid that if I counter him on it again he'll have me recalled, and there's too much valuable stuff to learn here to take that chance. I'm not kidding. Salvador and I are onto something big."

"*Qué?*"

"The cercariae begin to disappear from the water about four o'clock in the afternoon. We are guessing they won't return until about nine-thirty in the morning. How's that for banker's hours?" What do you suppose is behind that kind of periodicity?"

"Predation, my good friend. *Lebistes!* The little blighters that you plutocrats refer to as guppies, and buy for your tropical fish aquariums. You know what I mean?"

"Yes," I said. I was preparing to come in from the middle of the stream. Salvador had finished pumping.

"Thousands upon thousands of guppies. You've seen them near shore among the vegetation."

"Yes." I've often found myself caught up short, seeing in nature in the tropics thousands of a species of minnow or insect or snail that we buy for a dollar or two at the local pet shop in the States.

"It is in the literature. Just a casual 'one-liner.' I ran across it in the library at Tulane many years ago. I don't even remember the fellow's name. *Metcalf* maybe. China? I don't recall where he was working since I have never been as methodical as I should have liked to be. Too many irons in the fire. But because schisto is such a huge problem here, I used to routinely skim the abstract journals in the Tulane library every chance I got. I would do that even now if I were not confined to the *Espoleta.*

"And I have tested Metcalf's theory—let's call him Metcalf, anyway. One day I put a guppy in a beaker with a snail that was shedding cercariae. Twenty a minute at least; that translates into twelve hundred an hour. That's a bellyful if you ask me. Guppies are voracious predators!"

"You're kidding me," I said as I sloshed the last few feet to the bank. As I walked over to our folding camp table, Salvador held out the pizza pan and I centered the filter paper over a small pool of ninhydrin stain.

"I kid you not, *señor*. Believe me. It could explain your results with that contraption."

"Offhand, I'd say you could be right. If you are right, we have a powerful argument with which to stop the use of SCP. After all, we know the snails will be back in a matter of days. For the guppies it could take years."

"Harvey, you are a dreamer. It takes one to know one, believe me. The last thing Palma wants is to control schisto. That is what you do not understand about this business. With leprosy and yellow fever gone, with malaria more or less under control, he would lose the primary remaining source of his power base if he were to eliminate schisto. Schisto is his stepping-stone. He is banking his career on it. If anyone such as you tries to block him, he will likely turn nasty."

"He already has." I set the pizza pan containing the heat-dried filter paper aside next to the dissecting microscope. I couldn't talk and also study the paper accurately.

"Harvey, I am sure Emilia has told you that I majored in malariology in graduate school at Tulane. She may also have told you that I came home in July 1948 after earning my doctorate and that I worked for Palma for a couple of months. Emilia was already working at the lab under a clown named McBride, a grossly inferior *americano*. McBride left in a huff and Palma gave the job to Emilia. I don't think Palma knew that Emilia and I were very close friends.

"When I came home in '48, I had not seen her since high school in Comerio. However, even then in '48, we were both still incredibly young at heart and hopelessly idealistic. I can recall the many times that we talked practically through the night about what was wrong with the

Bucareli leadership; why Palma should never have been appointed Secretary of Health. Everywhere we saw worms in the woodwork—nepotism here, corruption there. Bucareli is a skunk; Palma, an accomplished crook. So how has anything changed?

"My visit in '48 lasted only for a few months. I did not stay long. I believed that with a bit more training I could play a constructive role in the Taviran legislature. So it was back to the United States to study political science and law in California.

"She is very astute, that Emilia. She could head the Department of Health so wonderfully. But Palma is a fox—more like a rabid fox. His mind was and is clearly on his advancement above all else, and he has planned accordingly."

"So it was in '48 that you tested the guppy predation report?"

"*Sí*. Only takes a minute to demonstrate. I am sure there are other predators, but guppies are convincing. Try it. You will be impressed."

"And then you returned in . . . in when?"

"June '51. Unfortunately, it soon became apparent that rather than politics and law in sunny California, I should have taken an intensive course of study at West Point."

I laughed. I was beginning to admire him. Apparently, he had reestablished his connection with Emilia after his return in '51.

"Harvey, we have an island here that needs to catch up with the century we live in. We have an economy based on sugar cane, a crop that will eventually lose out to sugar beets. We have rural workers worse off than your own coal miners were during The Great Depression. *Worse* off, mind you! They owe their children's souls, their grandchildren's souls, not just their own souls, to the company store, to *Centrale Allende*, that glistening diamond of the pre-industrial revolution. They owe the souls of their mothers and their sisters. All of them, every one of them is so far in debt he will go to the grave in debt. His children will go to the grave in debt. His grandchildren will go to the grave in debt.

"It has to stop. More accurately, it has to *be* stopped." He paused as though to see if I were paying attention. "I sound like your Ernie Ford, no?"

The same warm grin I'd seen him give Emilia spread across his almost boyish features. He looked about as much like a revolutionary as Bing Crosby.

"And who owns *Centrale Allende!*" he continued. "You have seen how the wealth has spread out from owner Bucareli to a wide range of his cronies. Do you think those people pay a fair share of taxes? *Centrale Allende* pays no taxes. The government subsidizes *Centrale Allende*. The government subsidizes sugar so that the price can be lower than the price of sugar from sugar beets.

"The wealth is here on Tavira, but it stays in some very special pockets. We are stuck with an immoral president, the teeth of whose dinosaur-based economy have severed a primary economic artery and are draining the last drops of blood from our treasury. We have an emasculated legislature. What a time in our history to also be stuck with a thief for a Secretary of Health."

I was about to say something in agreement when, suddenly, from behind him, I heard someone open the breach of a rifle and then slam a round into a chamber. It was the same alert that Emilia and I heard that day at the meadow high above Juncos where the snails bred in such huge numbers in the hoof prints of horses and cattle.

Abruptly Marcos melted into the darkness without another word. Perhaps his compatriots thought they heard an approaching vehicle. Perhaps they sensed some activity along the far side of the *Ebro*. I hoped they'd wait to find it was a false alarm.

GROUNDED

Salvador and I had guessed right. No cercariae appeared in the samples until 0900 hours. Of course we already knew that light stimulated cercarial release from the snails. Very likely, Marcos had provided the answer to our bigger question. Very likely, guppies gathered daily for a feed and decimated the cercarial population in the stream by late afternoon.

What a marvelously simple formula for halting transmission in the villages. Teach the villagers to use the water during the safe hours instead of in the noonday sun. Of course there might not be many takers for washing a load of clothes before breakfast or in the evening after dark. Still, there were plenty of inexpensive ways around that one once the villagers understood the problem and the need for a solution.

Over the ensuing weeks, Salvador and I repeated these hour-by-hour studies several times and in several places, always with the same results. I envisioned a huge educational program designed to spread the word amongst the rural population. With minor adjustments, rural villagers could live in the presence of schisto, and we would never ever need to treat the streams with chemicals. Eventually, transmission of the disease would fall below a magical threshold level and the disease would gradually disappear.

At the general staff meeting with Palma on the second of March, after Salvador and I were thoroughly convinced of the correctness of our data, I broke the news of our cercarial periodicity studies and I proposed putting our emphasis on an educational campaign rather than spraying to kill snails. Of course I did not let Palma know that we had done any of the work at Valencia. Valencia was far too valuable a property to lose.

Palma became enraged to learn that we had spent entire nights in the countryside without the army to protect us. "Marcos Díaz could have had you captured," he said. "He and his henchmen could have kidnapped you for ransom. Your stupid and foolhardy stunt could have cost the government millions of pesos in ransom. Or worse! You might have been murdered and the crime would forever reflect badly on Tavira. I forbid you to repeat such a idiotic act."

I glanced at Emilia. Our eyes met, but she gave no hint of her reaction to Palma's outburst. Within a week, Palma had given his order teeth. I soon found that I could not lease a vehicle anywhere on the Island. Make no mistake, a general ban such as that would have to be ordered by someone higher up than the boss of the Department of Health. No doubt, Palma got to Bucareli, and Bucareli laid down the law to every car rental agency on the Island.

Nor was that the end of it. Salvador and I soon found that even our daylight working hours had been trimmed. The Scout, we learned, could not be checked out until nine-thirty in the morning and had to be back by five in the afternoon. The shortened hours began to cut deeply into the productiveness of our research.

HOOF PRINT

Palma's new hours made it quite certain that a platoon of soldiers would show up to "protect" us on any *weekday* that we checked out the Scout and then worked at any of the sites that we had disclosed to Luis or to Palma. However, we found that we could easily get free of the soldiers with a little deception. We would pick a *disclosed* site and do a little routine post-treatment surveying. Then, we'd pack up the Scout, excuse the soldiers by telling them we were quitting early, and spend the rest of the day somewhere off the beaten track.

We soon learned another trick. The motor pool stayed open on weekends for the convenience of "senior" staff who might need a car for a weekend picnic or trip to the beach. It was a rank and privilege thing. I soon discovered that nothing prevented me from taking the Scout on Saturdays. Oddly, Palma's new restrictive hours applied to Saturdays, but Palma had not blocked my use of the Scout on Saturdays, and he had apparently not thought through the fact that the army worked a five-day week. Salvador loved the chance to work Saturdays. Hence, we discovered that we could be assured of this one day completely free of interference from the platoon of riflemen.

Apparently, few people were aware of the dirt and gravel road that could take us so easily from Valencia north through the forested ravines beside the *Segre*, then east past

Allende Cliff to the abandoned goldmine and to Hoof Print, the meadow where I first encountered Marcos.

Because we had an endless number of questions to answer relating to snail breeding at Hoof Print, Salvador and I were desperate to get up there as frequently as possible.

Of course, during these weeks, Palma did not yet have the funds to begin full-scale chemical control. Senator Pidal's bill to appropriate six million dollars was still "in committee." However, Palma was so eager to jumpstart his program that already he seemed to be trying to limit my activity to searching for places for him to treat with his deadly SCP.

Salvador and I decided to expand our own little game of cat and mouse, and also to make use of our Saturdays. First, I carefully explained to Palma that checking even two sites a day for infected snails would be the maximum that Salvador and I could do. I made the work seem time-consuming and complicated. Actually, we could easily check five or six streams a day, but I wasn't about to let Palma know that. Since he lacked sufficient experience with fieldwork to challenge my asserted limit of two sites, when things went right, we were able to work just a few hours a week for Palma and a whole bunch of hours for ourselves.

At least once a week, throughout the spring and early summer of 1959, Salvador and I would visit Hoof Print or downstream sites along the *Perico*. Marcos seemed irresistibly drawn to our studies at Hoof Print. Nearly always, as we parked the Scout and approached the meadow, he'd be there to meet us. He'd often spend the entire day with us helping to apply dabs of fast-drying, colored lacquer to the shells of snails. That was our most important preoccupation at Hoof Print itself. We'd mark five hundred snails the first of each month, and then search for them downstream the rest of the month. We often did find some of them downstream especially after a heavy rain. By using a different color each month, we obtained tremendously valuable data on movement of the snail population and on individual snail longevity.

One such day at Hoof Print was a Saturday, the Fourth of July. I was feeling a bit blue that morning, partly no doubt because of the restrictions Palma had us under, partly because the Fourth of July had always been my favorite holiday.

Usually, on the Fourth, as a child, I savored the trip to Burlington for the thrill of watching the parade—flags; marching high-school bands; often a new fire truck, its brass fittings beaming so brightly you could see your face in the huge nameplate on the driver-side door. Everyone seemed to enjoy the mayor's short and often comical tribute to our republic. I wondered that morning, as I shaved and dressed, how Salvador might handle such a day if, as mayor, he were put in charge of a similar celebration someday at a bigger, more fortunate Juncos.

I hurried through breakfast, ignoring the dull conversations of my *americano* tablemates as they discussed new prescription drugs and crop insecticides. As usual, the coffee was lukewarm and the toast lathered with cheap margarine. I signed the Scout out of the motor pool at exactly nine thirty.

I drove to *Centrale Allende* to fetch Salvador, arriving at ten fifteen. Salvador was waiting. Together, we reached Valencia at ten thirty and passed Allende Cliff about ten forty-five. No doubt Marcos's lookouts spotted us in the open woods as we passed the Allende Cliff turnoff, because Marcos was waiting for us as we walked onto the southern edge of Hoof Print about eleven thirty with all of our gear. In one hand Marcos held his rifle and in the other, a folding campstool.

Salvador and I set up our table on a patch of dry ground at the west side of the clearing. Marcos sat down across from me, while Salvador went off to collect the first of the five hundred snails that we planned to mark that day.

Marcos began a lengthy monologue as he meticulously prepared a workspace on his side of the small table.

"Harvey," he said, "when I was a youngster in high school in Comerio, our class was fortunate to have a really inspired biology teacher by the name of Soler, Justo Soler. God willing, I shall carry my memory of him to the grave. He had a great gray beard and an arthritic frame that must have pained him twenty-four hours a day. Emilia and I were both in that same biology class."

I detected a trace of desperation in Marcos's voice. I didn't see how it could stem from anything I'd said or done. I smiled and continued to arrange my workspace. Salvador was still collecting our first batch of snails. With five hundred snails to mark, and on our shortened schedule, this promised to be a busy day.

"I remember Justo Soler especially for his vivid tales of the campaign against yellow fever at the turn of the century," Marcos went on. "He promoted that wonderful epic in the history of tropical medicine into a tale that sang with emotion and intrigue: those wonderful experiments which proved Carlos Finlay right about mosquitoes transmitting the disease, and the courage of the United States Army volunteers who served as guinea pigs to prove that the virus could not spread directly from person to person. What a glorious age that was for tropical medical research. How could a man find a more soul-satisfying life? You have no idea how I envy you your work."

That *was* a "glorious age" in tropical medical research. The specialized and overlapping fields of medical entomology and parasitology that both Marcos and I had studied were born of that work in Cuba at the turn of the Century and evolved rapidly thereafter.

I brushed aside Marcos's envy regarding my occupation. "I'd say you're not doing badly yourself as careers go," I said. "Salvador thinks you're God's personal gift to Tavira."

He grinned just slightly. "But I also remember Justo Soler for another thing," he said. "Soler used to love to draw parallels from the *behavior* of different animal groups throughout the entire animal kingdom, both vertebrates and invertebrates. It made high school biology class so much more interesting than just dissecting dead frogs or watching the little brass arm of a flimsy old galvanometer inscribe its zigzag markings on the smoked paper on its drum. Remember those gadgets?"

"Yes," I said, realizing again how much Marcos and I had in common. Now, as I think back on those days and compare them with the much more complex stuff they teach today in high school and college biology, it seems incomprehensible that we have come so far so fast. I thoroughly agreed with Marcos that an inspiring teacher can influence a youth's entire life perhaps more than any other category of mentor.

I started to tell him of my own high school biology teacher, but Marcos was not accepting interjections. "I remember, too," he said, "Justo Soler's humorous tale about the mating behavior of crabs on a typical South American beach. Apparently, one cannot tell most of these crabs apart just by inspecting them from a distance. Even the crabs get confused from time to time. But they have developed a means of sorting themselves out.

"According to Soler, over centuries of inbreeding, each species has developed a collection of signals to help keep its members on the straight and narrow, so to speak. The males of each species wave their front claws, their chelicerae, in a special way. If a couple of crabs belonging to two different species start to approach each other with matrimony praying on their minds, the male will suddenly wave his chelicerae about in the air. The female, upon receiving an incorrect mating signal, will scurry away like a bear cub from a beehive.

"The male does not pursue her. He's not looking just for a bit of promiscuous fun, and he takes his responsibility to the species very seriously—much more seriously than a great many human beings, Soler might say.

"But here's the important part! Soler was quick to explain that in a stable, unvarying environmental situation, where conditions have remained the same for centuries—possibly for eons—there is a huge advantage to maintaining a homogeneous gene pool through carefully controlled inbreeding. In other words, if times are good, why 'rock the boat.' Or, as they say in California, 'Do not fix it unless it is broken.' Something like that. Maybe it's the other way around.

"As long as the environment remains stable, it is best for a well adapted species of animal to also remain genetically unchanged. Inbreeding is in; crossbreeding is out. That is how and why these 'chelicerae' mating signals evolved. Too much crossbreeding with another species of crab throws a monkey wrench into the gene pool that screws things up pretty fast."

Salvador had just supplied us with a great pile of snails to mark. The day was hot and the work far from done. Obviously, for a man with as active a mind as Marcos, this incredibly monotonous work fueled a compulsion to talk.

"However," he went on, "in an *unstable* environment, where conditions are beginning to change drastically, a highly inbred population soon finds itself in trouble, big trouble. Its members gradually lose the capacity to adapt. Something new comes along. Bam! They're gone. Their luck runs out. Like the dinosaurs. Well, no, maybe not quite like the dinosaurs . . ."

I began to wonder where all this was heading. I realized by that time that the desperation in his voice stemmed from the fear that he might not be able to hold my attention long enough to make his point, if there was one.

"Harvey, there are lessons to be learned from the behavior of those crabs on the beach that apply just as well to us as they do to crabs. Do we apply them? No!"

I shrugged and forced a smile.

"Exactly!" he said. "We tend to marry our own kind. No? Yes! However, even more significant than that, we drag these prejudicial patterns of behavior into every aspect of our lives. Conservatives elect conservatives; liberals, liberals. Monarchies appoint monarchs. Look at the French or the Russian Revolution. Both evolved from monarchies that had lost the capacity to adapt to change. In France, look how hard Turgot and those other two wizards of Louis XVI tried to initiate financial change in time and failed. The French government had become too inbred with upper crust in their fancy silks to meet the threat posed by the commoners.

"Or take Batista in Cuba. Same situation. Batista's cronies are rapidly losing the respect of a population disenchanted with gambling and corruption. Not even your Uncle Sam can keep Batista in power. Does your Uncle Sam have his finger in Tavira's pie as well?"

So that was it, I mused. "So that's the reason for the wallet-lifting exercise?" I said. "You thought I might be a secret agent from the States."

"Not I, Harvey. I hardly even knew you were coming to Tavira."

"Who then?"

He looked at me cautiously for an extended moment. Then he said, "The others will explain that to you someday. Leave it at that for now. I am sorry you were so offended by that wallet business."

I thought of asking him whom he meant by "the others," but instead I asked, "And when you've beaten the army and taken over the government, do you plan to use a guillotine on Bucareli, or will it be the firing squad?"

"That would be a joyous day! Too bad it could not happen today. Our two countries could share the same Fourth of July, no? Well, maybe next year. Do you remember your Fourth of July, Harvey? Do you remember *why* you have a Fourth of July; why the French gave you your Statue of Liberty?"

He looked down at his little pile of snails. I let it pass.

"I'd really prefer that you postpone your revolution until next year." I said. "I'll be finished with my work by then."

Marcos scowled. "Coward! So that is what you are." He turned to Salvador who hovered above us with a new bucket of snails. "Give the entire batch to Doctor Livingstone as punishment for poking fun at my enlightening lecture."

Salvador grinned and dumped the bucketful between us as usual.

With Salvador's superb assistance, Marcos and I managed, by three o'clock in the afternoon, to apply dabs of paint to the shells of close to five hundred snails. Salvador had collected the snails from the hoof prints using rubber gloves for protection. He'd brought them to us in batches ranging from fifty to a hundred. Marcos and I allowed the surface of the shells to dry in the sun just enough to accept the dab of colored lacquer, and then we returned them quickly to a container of fresh water.

Finally, Salvador, out of concern for the fragile habitat, carefully retraced his steps, gently placing snails at random into one hoof print or another.

Marcos and I had worked steadily. He *had* been unusually garrulous. I felt slightly embarrassed to have been such an indifferent listener. Marcos had spoken from the heart. Frankly, at the time, I recall that most of his message seemed a bit corny. Quaint, the thought of extrapolating from crab mating on a beach to Louis XVI.

Salvador hadn't said much all day. I doubt he'd caught much of our conversation. We drove in silence back to *Centrale Allende*. As he stepped down from the Scout at the gate to the factory, he said, "Tavira need very much Marcos Díaz, *doctor*. Please tell no one."

"*No problema*," I said.

I could tell that he liked my response. His conspiring expression conveyed his trust in me. I felt pretty good as I drove alone back to Aguilas to turn in the Scout at the motor pool. We'd made good use of our purloined day high up in the *Espoleta* beyond the reach of Palma and Bucareli's platoon of soldiers.

THE SHOOTERS

A tragedy occurred in mid-July. All spring and early summer, Palma had ordered, and Luis had faithfully carried out, the chemical spraying of a section of the *Perico* extending from its confluence with the *Rio Ebro* upstream for a distance of perhaps five hundred feet.

Meanwhile, at Juncos, Salvador and I collected snail repopulation data, determined the level of snail reinfection, and took daytime measurements of the number of cercariae per gallon of stream water. Keep in mind that Palma's insidious SCP had by now, killed all the guppies and other fish, the amphibians, and the insect larvae that had been present in abundance in the *Perico*. Snails, on the other hand, continued to wash downstream from Hoof Print and take up residence in quiet eddies along the length of the stream.

Many of these new snails were soon releasing cercariae, and we began to note horrendous surges in cercarial counts. The noon count at Juncos frequently rose to a hundred or more per gallon where once it had stabilized at a dozen or less. Even our last sample of the day taken at 4 P.M. showed these unusually high cercarial counts. Obviously, chemical treatment was doing more harm than good.

How we longed for an opportunity to continue overnight testing. I tried several times to explain to Palma the urgency of it. He would not relent.

With the guppy population decimated, Salvador and I thoroughly believed that we would have found cercariae in the water every hour of the day and night.

After Salvador and I had gathered all the useful data possible following an episode of SCP spraying, after snails had reestablished themselves and cercarial levels had stabilized, I would step into Palma's office and tell him that Juncos was again a hot spot. That approach and timing reinforced Palma's belief that Salvador and I were cooperating. Usually, even as I stood before his desk, Palma would lift the telephone handset and order Luis to spray the *Perico*. Usually the very next day, Luis would go to Juncos with a small crew, his two backpack sprayers, and the dregs of the dwindling supply of SCP. The chemical was appallingly expensive. Apparently, Palma had decided not to order more until Senator Pidal's appropriation bill came out of committee and was voted into law.

As I've said, Luis and I were under orders to notify Palma whenever we planned to take a crew into the field. When we notified Palma, he passed the word on to the army base and the base sent a team of ten riflemen under the command of a corporal to "protect us" in case by some miracle the guerrillas should decide to show up. Of course, we didn't need the protection. Hence, Salvador and I often played forgetful. Not so Luis. With a family to support, he consistently towed the line.

On Friday, July 17, about noon, the soldiers were deployed along the stream at Juncos. The spray team was spraying. Salvador and I were packing up our gear after gathering some last minute data. We hadn't expected the sprayers to arrive until afternoon.

Suddenly, in the quiet of that hot summer day, Salvador's grandson, Hernando García, a skinny eighteen year old, home on vacation from his first year at the Agricultural College at Comerio, crossed under one of the footbridges that spanned the stream and stepped out of the shadows into the sun. He was on his way to greet his grandfather. Unfortunately, he held a half-foot length of sugar cane in one hand. Possibly, to the untrained eye, the stubby length of cane, partly blackened by mildew, might have passed for a weapon of some kind, but no experienced soldier would be likely to misread it.

Apprehensively, I looked quickly from Hernando to the nearest riflemen and I caught a quick exchange of glances between two of the soldiers. My heart sank as one gave a nod of approval. The two fired simultaneously and Hernando staggered back against the foundation of the bridge. Salvador reached him before he could fall, embracing him even as blood poured from his chest. I stood stunned as the bloodied water cut a crimson swath that spread downstream toward the boot of the closest shooter. Then, as my faculties returned, I charged across the stream to help Salvador.

Together, we lifted Hernando to dry ground and laid him gently on a bed of fallen blossoms shed from an aging balsa that shaded the west side of the bridge.

Salvador turned briefly to catch the eye of one of the assailants. I shall never forget the hatred in that stare. Then he turned again quickly to tend to Hernando.

"*No entiendo!*" were the only faint words Hernando was able to speak as he died. He seemed at peace, not frightened or in pain. He whispered the words twice.

Gently, Salvador closed Hernando's eyelids, and then wordlessly, we exchanged a lingering glance. I knew at that moment that our fabulous experience of working together was over.

There was no way I could console Salvador; we both were coping with too much anger to be of use to one another. News travels fast along the banks of mountain streams. A hostile crowd began to gather. Tension mounted and the soldiers staged a tactical retreat towards the truck as the angry villagers, mostly women, closed in. Had the husbands been home from the cane fields there most certainly would have been more bloodshed.

I sought out the corporal in charge. By the time I got his attention I was too angry to think. Finally, I blurted out, "What were your orders?"

"To shoot anyone with gun."

"Are you all blind?" I shouted.

"It look like pistol," he said unconvincingly.

"Cane? Thick as your wrist? What kind of pistol would that be? A pirate's blunderbuss? A youth with your country's college logo on his T-shirt?"

Luis joined us. "Sooner or later it was bound to happen," he said.

"That's not an excuse," I growled.

"I know it's not an excuse," he said meekly.

I wanted to grab Luis by the neck and shake some backbone into him. I was coping with that compulsion when the corporal abruptly mounted the running board, climbed into the passenger's seat next to the driver, and slammed the door in our faces. The driver backed the truck around and they sped off to the east along the *Ebro*.

"Damn you, Luis," I said, "why don't you just once try to stand up for something? You've only got one life. Use it!"

"Well, if they come out here with their guns, sooner or later they're going to use them."

"That was no case of 'sooner or later!' I saw one nod to the other two seconds before they fired."

He said nothing. Yet he didn't look away. He simply stared at me in a most disheartened way, and his expression brought me to my senses. I had no business cursing him when his world held so much less hope and comfort and security than my own.

"Did Palma request the platoons," I asked, "or did Bucareli insist on them?"

"They were Bucareli's idea. I doubt Palma was given a choice," Luis said. "Do you remember Emilia's question at that meeting?"

"Partially." I said. "She tried to tell Palma that the guerrillas might not take kindly to spraying the creeks and streams in the *Espoleta.* Palma turned sarcastic and told her Bucareli was already on top of that possibility."

"Do you recall that in addition to sending the squads of riflemen Palma also said at that meeting that Bucareli planned to attack the guerrillas in force?"

"Yes."

"If that happens, your work and mine will be over." His voice betrayed his emotion. "It could be a long siege. No one knows how strong Marcos Díaz is in terms of men and matériel. It is possible that he could give the army quite a beating and hold out a long time in the *Espoleta.*"

I still felt stunned and almost sick to my stomach. I looked back towards the footbridge. Salvador had disappeared.

"It is a sad thing and a very bad thing," Luis said. "However, I will say again that it was bound to happen sooner or later. There was no reason to send troops to guard my sprayers. We have never been in danger. Palma knows that. Bucareli knows that. Most Department of Health employees, like Salvador, grew up in these villages. They have family and friends here. They would not ever be in danger from the guerrillas."

We stood together a moment longer near his truck, surveying the scene. Then Luis said, "Harvey, I want you to know that I agree with you. Spraying is the wrong way to control schisto. At least in the long run. In fact, many in the department feel as you do. And the facts you and Salvador have uncovered about the daily presence of cercariae in the water have brought many others over to your side. Clearly the data suggest new, important ways of attacking the disease."

"Then why haven't you stated these beliefs and this growing support in our meetings with Palma?"

"It would do no good."

"You don't know that until you try it. He has to know what his staff thinks. That's the way it's supposed to work. It's the only way it *can* work."

"Palma already understands fully the significance of your cercarial studies, Harvey. Palma is the Secretary of Health. I am not in charge. And I have grandchildren who, like Hernando, dream of college. But mine hope to attend college in the United States. That costs, as you say in America, big bucks. Every day I tell myself, *hang in there, Luis*. Maybe, if I can do that, without accidentally hanging myself in the process, mine can realize their dreams. That would make my wife so very happy, so very proud. So then, how do I balance that with the killing of a few fish in the *Perico* and the other streams?"

"It won't be just a few fish, Luis, not after Pidal's appropriation passes."

"I'm sorry, but my priorities and Tina's happiness will always be the determining factor in my decisions."

I looked at him with surprise. I realized that I had never heard him speak her name. "Tina must be a lovely person," I said. What else could I say? When a sleeping, traditional, agricultural economy begins to stir, there seems to be a sort of early pause along the way where the dreams of the disadvantaged surface to hinder the process. I'd seen it happen before Tavira, and in many places later on in my career. Sometimes, even to tempt change seems cruel, so many are hurt or disappointed along the way. Yet, to leave half the world hamstrung by poverty and disease can only lead to a disparity of ever more dangerous proportions.

I remembered noticing while in Tanzania that personalities seemed much more transparent than at home. The same was true on Tavira. Perhaps the pace of change causes this to be so. There are always the movers and shakers, the utterly secure, persistent risk takers usually from amongst the privileged, but there are legions of the cautious, like Luis, for whom job security looms larger than any other goal. The latter have not yet seen proof that there will still be work to do after they complete the work they've been assigned. Luis was clinging to the first good job he'd ever had. I had no right to ask him to risk it.

I looked around to see if Salvador had returned. He'd gone with the villagers who'd carried Hernando's body home. My heart ached for him. He'd been so proud and spoke so often of Hernando—so much promise wiped out in an instant.

Luis left me and worked his way upstream along the bank. He spoke to several villagers along the way, and returning to say that Salvador wanted to remain with the body. Then Luis called in his crew of sprayers, and ordered them to load the truck. Still dazed by the events of the day, I watched as they gathered up their things.

They were nearly done when Luis returned to my side and said completely out of nowhere, "Harvey, I am envious of your independence in this work we are doing. You have 'the courage of your convictions.' I admire that. We need your example. Your example may be the most important thing you give us." Then he pulled himself up into the front seat of the truck beside the driver.

For a moment, his last remark carried me two thousand miles north to my childhood home in Vermont. My mother used to have a cartoon pasted on her refrigerator door. I think she'd clipped it from an old *New Yorker* magazine. It pictured two sturdy women watching their young sons pass by as part of a Fourth of July parade. One was saying to the other, "Look, everybody is out of step but my Willie!" I don't know why, but I described the cartoon to Luis as the truck prepared to leave. I don't think he knew how to take it. He came as close as I'd ever seen him come to producing a smile. But it faded just as quickly. He signaled his driver to move on.

Many times, on my visits to home as a young man, I read the caption to that cartoon without perceiving more than the simple message that possibly aptitude played a part in Willie's limited success at close-order drill. But, with age, I came to realize that some of us are out of step by choice, our reasons as diverse as the constellations we contemplated in our youth on clear summer nights as we lay beneath a universe of stars.

POWER AND POLITICS

Emilia was heartbroken over the death of Hernando. Not surprisingly, I learned that she had been one of several who recommended him for a scholarship at the Agricultural College at Comerio.

"How is Salvador taking it?" she asked me some days later as I was leaving the building on my way to the motor pool.

"I don't know. I haven't seen him since that fateful Friday," I said.

"Isn't he showing up for work?"

"Not so far this week. Before the shooting, we'd planned that I would pick him up at the *centrale* gate each day so we could work the streams west of Valencia. It saves a lot of time if I meet him there. I've stopped and waited each day, but he doesn't show."

"And today?"

"I'll try again."

"I mean, what's on for today?"

"A short day at Valencia."

"Did you turn in a trip report to Palma for today?"

"Do you mean will the guard platoon be waiting at Valencia?"

"Yes."

"No. I'm not being very cooperative about that."

"Have you been to Juncos since it happened?"

"No."

"Why not?"

"Frankly, I don't have the nerve. I feel somehow responsible."

"Let me go with you today. But only if you will agree to stop at Juncos just for a moment? He could be staying with his daughter, Francesca. Perhaps I can talk to him. Work might help him handle his grief."

"Whether he's there or not, I have to get some work done at Valencia."

"How long will you need at Valencia?"

"A couple of hours."

"Okay, then there is plenty of time. First we look for Salvador at Juncos, then at the *centrale* gate, then we go on to Valencia. If we find him, you and he do what you need to do at Valencia and then plan your next workday. Then we drop him off at the *centrale* and you and I drive back to Aguilas."

"That's basically okay except we'll be late meeting up with Salvador if he *is* waiting at the *centrale* gate."

"Well, if he has caused you delay every day this week, he can hardly complain."

She followed me to the motor pool, and settled herself into the passenger's seat of the Scout with no further affirmation from me. As we drove out of the motor pool and got underway, she commented that Hernando's killing could not have happened at a worse time, and in a worse place and way.

"That's an understatement," I said.

She turned towards me. "So two of them fired?" she said.

"Yes, almost simultaneously."

"So you do not view it as an accident or the result of poor or inadequate training?"

"No way. In fact, it's worse than that."

"How do you mean?"

"Hernando emerged from the darkness under the little foot bridge, but he did not look menacing in any way that I could see. He carried a short, thick stick of sugar cane in one hand. The corporal made the excuse afterward that it looked like a pistol."

"But you are having trouble with that?" she interrupted.

"Yes."

"How come?"

"Because I happened to notice an interaction between the two shooters. They glanced at each other. Then the one who was closest gave a little nod the way you might say 'let's do it' to someone with whom you have a prior agreement."

"You're certain?"

"I know what I saw."

Emilia was silent for more than a minute, and then she said, "Did you sense at all that Marcos was around Juncos at thc time."

"No."

"Do you know what I think?" she said. "I think Bucareli ordered a shooting as a way of discrediting Palma with the villagers. Look at it this way: if it appears Palma's program is bringing danger to the villagers, he will be unable to win rural votes. I think Bucareli has figured out that Palma can beat him in the January elections." She paused for a moment, and then her mood changed. "I've got to get a message to Marcos today. I can take care of that at Juncos. It will only take a few minutes."

I glanced at her. She was really taking me into her confidence. And apparently she was thoroughly mixed up in this thing. I decided to try her further. "What kind of mcssage?"

She studied me for a moment, her lips slightly parted and just a trace of a smile on her face. "Oh, some supplies he ordered have arrived. He needs to make arrangements to pick them up at the warehouse."

"What sort of supplies?"

"Ammunition. Rifle rounds. Ten cases. I think they'd fit nicely in the Scout." She sat there looking at me rather casually.

"Holy cow, Emilia! Don't put something like that on me!"

"It would not be much out of your way."

I looked at her with total disbelief, and very nearly ran the Scout off the shoulder.

She folded her arms beneath her breasts, and began to laugh. "I am so sorry, Harvey. I could not resist. I wanted to see how you would react."

"You frightened me terribly. I was thinking *what in Sam Hill kind of a mess have I gotten myself into, talking sedition, planning to tote arms for a revolutionary in the hills?* So what part of this tale is true? Is there any ammo to be delivered?"

"I just couldn't resist. You looked so funny and serious. Do you know how funny you look when you are especially serious?"

I ignored her remark. "Do you even have a message to deliver to Marcos?"

"Heavens no! Marcos is too old-fashioned to put me in harm's way. I'm supposed to use 'the alternative message route,' remember."

Then her thoughts seemed to turn inward, a mood I'd observed many times. "I wish it were otherwise," she said.

"What *otherwise*? What are we talking about?"

"I would love to be part of his private little revolution. I would rather be up there cooking for him or mending his socks than down here having to put up with Palma."

"Well, you're needed down here just now. Marcos can mend his own socks." My sudden sense of envy surprised me. I realized that it hadn't gone unnoticed. I changed the subject abruptly. "By the way, speaking of supplies and warehouses, Charlie Bauer wouldn't have anything to do with supplying Marcos, would he?"

She didn't hesitate a moment. "If I knew, I wouldn't tell you."

"I didn't think you would."

"But I will tell you this much, and I shouldn't. Charlie Bauer is responsible for your pocket being picked."

"What do you mean?"

"He ordered it."

"Who ordered him to order it?"

"Nobody. He does it on his own. Or at least it seems that way."

We had cleared the city and were heading north.

"What's his motivation?" I asked.

"Nobody seems to know. He has been doing it for several years. Nothing is ever stolen from the wallets. The police never seem to have enough proof to arrest him. And they would not arrest him anyway. I'm told that he reports his findings from these little escapades directly to Bucareli.

"Furthermore, he is too important to the economy. He has too many connections. He can get things for Bucareli and his gang of thieves that no local importer would ever be able to get. And he gets them fast. If you want a new foreign car, say a convertible with red leather seats, all you need to do is ask Charlie. He has a catalog room. Wealthy housewives spend days in there ordering everything from refrigerators to window drapes to the latest styles in furniture and clothing."

"Do you remember, up at the meadow that day, when I blamed Marcos for having my wallet lifted?"

"Yes. I thought it silly that you did that. Why would Marcos know about that?"

"You think he didn't? He certainly knew my wallet had been stolen. Remember his reply? *Pinned that on me, did you?* Remember that?"

"Yes, I do. And it interests me that you can repeat things people say word for word. How do you do that?"

"Do what?"

"Repeat things word for word."

"I don't know. Attention to detail, I guess. How a person words something is usually more important than the message itself. My point is that if Charlie ordered it and Marcos knew about it—"

"And I'm supposed to conclude that Charlie works for Marcos—"

"Or Marcos works for Charlie. Wouldn't that be something?"

"Harvey, stop this! Don't even think it."

"It's possible that both Charlie and Marcos find it prudent to monitor arrivals from the States that might impact them in some way. Bucareli could be importing some of those U.S. 'advisors.' Something like that."

"Masquerading as preoccupied scientists? Awfully far-fetched." She was gazing out the car window. We passed a lovely row of tamarind trees just off the shoulder of the road. The bare ground beneath the tamarinds seemed swept with a broom. Beyond them, a fence-line clothed with the rosy blossoms of coralita separated the tamarinds from a sea of yearling sugar cane.

We crossed the *Ebro* at the shallow point where Salvador and I first crossed that June day thirteen months ago. The water was not too high and the gravel beneath our tires seemed firm. Tavira had been unseasonably dry that spring.

When we reached Juncos, Emilia left me to go up towards Salvador's house. She was gone at least an hour. I waited impatiently in the Scout.

She returned to the Scout with the news that Salvador had quit his job with the Department of Health. He'd sent his note of resignation with the school bus driver the Monday after the shooting. Emilia said that he'd blamed his resignation on his age and poor health. Perhaps that fooled Palma, but I'm sure it fooled no one at Juncos.

I asked her if she had actually talked with Salvador. She didn't answer the question directly. She would only say that Salvador would arrange to work with me later on, not right away.

I sensed that Salvador was not up there at his shanty or his daughter's shanty. Had he been there, I think he'd have walked down to talk with me. We knew each other far too well to need to converse through an intermediary, even one as amiable as Emilia, even in his grief.

From Juncos, Emilia and I retraced our route back to the shallow gravel crossing and then west along the south side of the *Ebro* to Allende Bridge. After a brief wait at the gate of the *centrale*, we reached Valencia shortly after noon.

Emilia visited a dwelling or two, but she spent most of the hour by my side as I did my snail count. I wanted to run some other tests, but decided to forego them until the following week.

We headed for home at about 2:30, and on the way, Emilia brought up again the murder of Hernando.

"Our speculation is correct as to why Hernando was killed," she said.

"How do you know?"

"You mentioned that you noticed the exchange between the two shooters, the glance, the nod?"

"Yes."

"I learned at Juncos that those two men were added to the guard platoon at the last minute by orders from way up above. They were two of Bucareli's most trusted bodyguards. Isn't that just about the most disgusting thing you can imagine?"

"Yes." I felt my anger returning.

"In Juncos, the villagers believe as I do that Bucareli arranged the shooting to discredit Palma. Palma stood to gain a lot of supporters in the villages of the *Espoleta* if he played his cards right, especially if he got the people to like him, if they believed him to be genuinely interested in their welfare."

"Who told you this?"

For a moment, she didn't answer. Then she said, "Actually, it was Marcos. Marcos learned about the bodyguards from a confederate he has within the military." Her voice broke as she spoke. "They are so cruel and evil. To feed their dirty political ambitions they kill a youth without the slightest compunction."

For a moment, I didn't take my eyes off the road. I could tell she was almost in tears. My own vision was blurred with emotion. I pulled over onto the shoulder and took her in my arms, and she wept on my shoulder. "What is so wonderful about being the leader that makes you men kill for it?"

I had no answer to give her.

A MOST DIFFICULT TASK

Friday July 24, Emilia, Luis, Gregorio, and I were seated as usual about the little alcove in Palma's office. His secretary, José Carrera, had let us in and provided us with coffee. José was a solemn, negative, unpleasant fellow with more the build of a line blocker than a quarterback. In fact, his fingers were so thick I don't see how he managed a standard typewriter or carried a coffee cup by its handle.

We'd been seated in the alcove for at least fifteen minutes when Palma finally strode in.

"Get ready to work hard," he ordered as he moved directly to his desk.

We realized immediately that this meeting was to have a different setting, and we began to arrange chairs for ourselves opposite his desk.

"I shall assume that you all know by now that Pidal's appropriation bill passed the Senate late yesterday afternoon. As of this morning we have a huge budget to review, and a division of labor to assign."

Nothing was said initially about the death of Hernando. It certainly was not to be first on his agenda. But I guessed from his especially cold attitude towards me that he would eventually bring it up. Out there at Juncos, I'd let the corporal know I was angry, and the word on that may have gotten back to Palma indirectly.

"Our title for the new project," he went on, "for correspondence, public relations, news releases, and all other contacts will be *Terreno Difícil* to honor the fact that we are embarking on a hard road never walked before—the total annihilation of a single species of snail from an entire land mass."

I must admit that Palma had style. Under different circumstances, I might have liked him. I certainly had to respect his bureaucratic skills even while I found nothing in my heart but contempt for his brand of science.

"Gregorio has agreed to act as purchasing agent for the project in addition to his regular duties. Emilia, Luis, and even you, Harvey, will requisition your supplies through him using our special project forms. On the first round or two of big orders that each of you will be making, I suggest you search the catalogues over at Charlie Bauer's and then clear your choices through Gregorio. In turn, he will obtain my approval or rejection before actually placing the orders. In addition to supervising all purchase orders, Gregorio will handle all invoices and payrolls. He will continue to do payrolls for our regulars as well as the new staff that we will be hiring."

Actually, there was nothing new about the forms that Palma referred to. Only the title, *Terreno Difícil,* was new. We'd coped with drafts of these newly proposed forms over the last few weeks. They'd crossed our desks on a daily basis. No doubt, Palma ate, slept, and paced his office with his dreams for this new project.

"Luis will have the most work to do. On his shoulders rests the responsibility for outfitting the new trucks and purchasing backpack sprayers and other equipment. On his shoulders also rests the responsibility for selecting and employing most of the new personnel. I must approve all of his decisions. Recruiting, alone, represents an enormous assignment. Altogether, remember, we are looking at fifty spray trucks and about two hundred new field men."

I could hardly believe the man's ludicrous grasp of the realities of the fieldwork. There was no way Luis could monitor fifty teams in the field full time, and it would take years to find and train enough men to adequately supervise so much detailed work.

"I have decided that our base of operations for the project will be at the old leprosy compound at Corejo. Luis will need to organize and equip those facilities to suit our needs. Initially, that will require teams of carpenters, electricians, plumbers, and other subcontractors.

"Luis will help Gregorio find the least expensive source of supply for SCP. When it arrives, Luis will oversee its storage. We already know the stuff is costly. Its supervision is a major responsibility. I am told that it must be kept dry and in a well ventilated area."

Actually, he had that about half right. Concentrated SCP is a severe irritant and can be absorbed through the skin to cause extensive damage to the body. It is also extremely unstable when stored as a powder rather than in solution. If it reaches its flashpoint, it decomposes violently, leaving little residue. Once, while in Tanzania, I had to supervise the disposal of about five pounds of it. Quite a sight. Palma was talking half-a-ton.

"Emilia, you have your own responsibilities," he continued. "You will be running two laboratories simultaneously. All laboratory work for *Terreno Difícil* will be done at Corejo. You will have to divide your time effectively between Corejo and here. In addition to setting up the Corejo lab, I expect you to assist Luis by interviewing workers who apply for Luis's openings as well as your own and Harvey's. You should go out to the sites with Luis on occasion so that you can understand thoroughly the nature of the work his men are required to do."

Adapting the old Corejo barracks for specialized fieldwork would be a challenge. I knew Emilia would do a masterful job of it. But it would be hard work. She'd need proper lab benches, centrifuges, and gas jets—the works.

"You should also spend sufficient time in the field with Harvey to understand how he does his post-treatment surveys. We will need one post-treatment crew of five men to work with Harvey and we will get Harvey some sort of delivery truck. Does that suit you, Harvey?"

I shrugged and said that I supposed that would work. I envisioned myself spending every moment of my remaining months on Tavira tooling about the island with five men in a square van, like a furniture store driver with nothing to deliver but evidence that Palma's beloved *Terreno Difícil* had proven too *difícil.* However, I was happy that Emilia would be allowed to accompany me at least in the early stages of the program.

Surprisingly, Palma eventually invited questions and we spent several hours that day, and for the next several working days, going over the details.

Nothing about that first meeting pleased Emilia more than to have permission to join me in the field. It came as an unexpected bonus. She had a virtual license to engage in treason, shuttling messages and perhaps even small weapons and equipment to Marcos on the pretense of observing my post-treatment methodology.

Apparently, Palma was in too good a mood to want to dwell on the subject of Hernando's death. "So you need a new primary field man?" he said to me as the meeting ended.

"Oh, I think I can get Salvador to work with me from time to time on a volunteer basis," I said.

"Well, that will be fine for now if you can swing it. Maybe after the chemical arrives and we get going on the spraying in a big way we can find a permanent replacement for him."

I thanked him. It was immaterial. Nobody could replace Salvador.

Palma turned again to Luis. "I know it isn't any fault of yours that the boy was killed. The youth had no business lurking around in the dark under that foot bridge—not with riflemen about."

Luis's expression was that of the perfect subordinate. "You are probably right," he said. "However, the tragedy will impact our work. It is going to be difficult to work at Juncos. The villagers were openly hostile. And news travels fast in the *Espoleta*."

"That is a fact," Gregorio said.

"Exactly," Emilia joined in. "I'm sure every community in the foothills knows about it by now."

Palma gauged their unanimity. "Nobody ever promised that this would be an easy project to carry out. On the contrary!"

I wish I'd had the nerve to quip that nothing's easy that's flawed from the start.

"I suppose Salvador's sudden retirement is related to Hernando's death?" Palma asked.

"It may have hastened it somewhat," I said. "But he'd confided in me numerous times that he planned to retire soon." I lied. "And I've noticed this last month that he's mighty short of breath sometimes." Actually, Salvador could have run circles around me any day of the week. He loved the work. It brought him a sense of giving back to his villagers something that could benefit them for generations to come. Now there was no conceivable way he could work for me again on a regular basis, especially at Juncos.

I knew I would see Salvador again, but I could never have guessed the circumstances.

THE PLANETARY IMPACT

Salvador or no Salvador, I had to mark the August batch of five hundred snails at Hoof Print, so, on Wednesday, August 5, I set out alone. It was a hot, wet, muggy, summer day and the mountain road from Valencia up along the *Segre* was eroded and treacherous. Without the 4-wheel drive I could never have made it even halfway.

When I finally arrived at the abandoned mine, I parked the Scout as usual beneath a group of giant mountain gommier trees that seemed to reach halfway to heaven, stretching their massive trunks far above the lower canopy of figs, tree ferns, and a thousand other native species.

Although it was a short walk to Hoof Print from the mine, I carried my marking kit and Salvador's gloves, containers, and bottles of isopropyl alcohol. I'd need to do both his work and mine.

Marcos was there to greet me when I arrived. He stood dead center amongst the breeding snails with each foot in a hoof print.

"I know what you are thinking," I said. "You expect me to exclaim, aghast, that you are exposing yourself to infection. Then you will be able to brag about how carefully you instruct your men not to pollute the water and infect the snails here in the breeding ground or elsewhere."

"You are right, Amigo. You are not an easy one to fool. You could at least play along with me. This has been a humorless day thus far." He headed towards the patch of dry ground where I usually set up my small worktable.

"And what makes today so grim?" I asked.

"Today I learned more details of *el señor* jackass Palma's outrageous plan. Fifty vehicles! Preposterous!"

"Did you hear about the depot at Corejo?"

"Yes. And *you* my friend; I fear your research days are over. He has you doing nothing but the post-treatment surveys. What joy could you possibly find in that?"

"None. But I can do his work and still sneak some time for basic research. I could do the basic research a lot faster if you hadn't stolen Salvador away."

"I am sorry, *señor.* He came of his own freewill. Of course I offered him substantially higher rank and pay than the Department of Health would ever have paid him. He is my new supply officer. At the present time, he is at the very north tip of the Island where the *Espoleta* meets the sea, inventorying our supplies."

Until that day, I had no concept of the strength of Marcos's forces. Certainly, Bucareli's lieutenants knew nothing of the huge ordinance Marcos had amassed. However, that day, as we dabbed five hundred snails with dots of colored lacquer, Marcos, described the tons of supplies carefully stashed away in a dozen huge natural caves along the north coast of the *Espoleta.*

"And I suppose," I said, "that you order this stuff from some sort of gunrunner's catalog and the postman delivers it?"

With his toothpick, Marcos arranged a dozen snails into a neat row and paused to let the sun dry their cumbersome coiled shells. "If Charlie Bauer had not prearranged the picking of your pocket on the plane, if Emilia had not tested your timbre and found you trustworthy, if Salvador had not vouched for you, and I myself had not seen you with my own eyes midstream in the *Segre* in the middle of the night holding the end of a garden hose like some mother's idiot *muchacho*, do you think for a moment I would be sitting here revealing the details of over five years of desperate hopes and plans?

"Charlie has the catalogs in a special concealed cabinet. Best of all, his suppliers make the deliveries direct to the north coast beaches. They anchor offshore at night beyond the coral reefs and send the stuff in on lighters with less draft than a native dugout canoe.

"Those same reefs make attack from the north a near impossibility. Without amphibious landing craft, which Bucareli doesn't have, his soldiers would face withering fire if they approached on lighters or tried to wade on foot over the coral.

"It is good, solid logistics. We have sort of a bucket-brigade system for moving ammunition and canned food from the northern caves to the defensive positions on the south side of the *Espoleta*, where most of us are quartered."

"So," I said, "you had to have the help of my best friend, an eighty year old man, to count all this stuff? You don't have anyone else capable of keeping track of the inventory?"

"Oh, Harvey, surely you know I didn't draft him. You could see with your own eyes what Hernando's murder did to him."

I smiled. "I'm kidding. Of course I understand." I asked him if he knew that Bucareli had issued orders for an attack.

"Yes, and they are in for a surprise."

"Are you sure they don't know the extent of your ordinance?"

"Not according to my informants. Bucareli assumes that my supplies come in through the villages of Juncos, Valencia, and two other communities along the south rim of the *Espoleta*, that we are armed with rifles and a few rounds of ammunition. The difficulty we face is that once we go on the offensive we cannot withdraw back into the safety of the *Espoleta*. If we do, Bucareli will certainly subject the villagers to brutal retribution. Once the battle is joined, we have to rally the general population to our cause. We *must* win. Perhaps more than any other factor, this responsibility towards the villagers has kept us from engaging in guerrilla tactics that could have gradually depleted Bucareli's army.

"Yet, sooner or later, something has to give. Charlie cannot keep on providing us with supplies forever. Eventually he'll be found out. Time is not on his side. With revolution, as with all things, there is a moment when one must act with dedication and passion or choose not to act at all."

He had been fiddling nervously with a new row of snails, arranging them first one way and then another like a platoon of new recruits. Finally, he dipped the end of his toothpick in the lacquer and placed a drop of color on first one and then another. The color for August was robin's egg blue.

I hoped, unlike our previous meeting at Hoof Print on the Fourth of July, that I might be spared a heavy dose of his homespun philosophy. No such luck.

"You know what, Harvey, humans are pack animals. Dogs are pack animals. Wolves are pack animals. Hyenas are pack animals. Baboons are pack animals . . . even chimps are sort of pack animals."

"How are you defining *pack animals*?"

"They establish a hierarchy through tribal contests for dominance. They tend to have only one leader at a time. They assign him inordinate powers. Any member can challenge a leader, and, if deposed, the leader is either killed or forced to leave the pack—exiled. Primitive, no? Yes!

"Surely, you have seen some of those museum-case, panoramic scenes of wooly, early man attacking an equally wooly mammoth. We may have been pack animals since the beginning of time."

"This has a familiar ring to it," I said.

"Not exactly."

"So we are not remounting your *adaptation* hobby-horse?"

"Absolutely not."

"We're not back to Louis XVI and the waving chelicerae?"

"Definitely not!"

"Or Batista in Cuba?"

"No, not really. Napoleon and Hitler are better examples of the point I have in mind."

"That won't wash," I pointed out. "Napoleon and Hitler were not deposed by members of the pack. They were driven from power by members of other packs."

"It is not important. The pack merely expanded temporarily. The important thing is to note that as humans we establish hierarchies and pick individual leaders whom we tend to worship or to humiliate. We do this in politics. We do this in religion. We do this with our entertainers and our movie stars. You, in America, do this even with your beauty queens . . . although I see signs that you are growing out of that infantile pattern."

Without Salvador to collect snails for us to mark, the new Marcos monologue was repeatedly interrupted as I made trips among the hoof prints either to collect or release snails. On the previous visit, the Fourth of July, the work had gone twice as fast. However, this month, had Marcos not helped, I doubt I could have gotten the job done at all. Even so, since Marcos preferred talking to painting, it promised to be a long day.

"You may notice another interesting thing about the pack-animal phenomenon," he said. "The tenure differs.

Politicians and religious leaders, once given the right to lead, usually get the most time to prove themselves. Movie stars and vocalists reign for a medium term. Revolutionaries are given a longevity almost as short as that of standup comics."

As I returned another batch of freshly marked snails to the hoof prints, it occurred to me, *God forbid if snails should also be pack animals.* Here, we had removed a whole bunch of well adjusted little packers from their native hoof prints, mixed them up, and then plunged them at random right into the territorial domains of rival packs. We could be accused of creating snail social chaos, of causing multiple neuroses, of instilling every kind of stress imaginable.

As our work ended that day, I began to collect my things. It was then that Marcos made a point I shall always remember him for.

"Curiously, the political leaders that humans have selected over the millennia resemble the leaders that typical pack-animal species select. We pick them for their muscles rather than their minds. More often than not, they are strong and egotistical. Occasionally, they are ruthless and cunning. We do not seem to bother to take the time to define the job description of a leader in such a way as to enhance our chance of selecting a *true* leader. And over the centuries we have found ways to rid ourselves of hundreds of *true* leaders. The cream of the crop in the human pack have been nailed to the cross, forced to drink hemlock, excommunicated by the church, and condemned at the voting poles. In their stead, we almost invariably pick the worst of the pack to lead us."

"So you are saying that our frame of reference vis-à-vis what constitutes leadership is not so hot?"

"Exactly! Crabs that cannot adapt; baboons that cannot lead—*todo me es igual!* It makes no difference. The big question is not what is best for *this* nation or *that* nation, or *this* religion or *that* religion, or *this* industry or *that* industry. We need to learn to challenge every human decision with just one question: How will this decision effect the health and longevity of our planet?"

Quite perceptive for the 1950s—but I recall saying, "You'd never get support for a fanciful idea like that."

"Amigo, for shame," he said lightheartedly, "you are such a pessimist."

For a while, after I'd finished packing my things, we discussed Hernando's death and the impact it would have on Palma's program of snail eradication. I shared with him what I knew of Palma's plans. He rejoiced to learn that Emilia had been given free license, at least for the time being, to accompany me to stream sites in the *Espoleta*.

As Salvador had said, "Tavira need very much Marcos Díaz." I wondered as I drove back to Aguilas if his little band of guerrillas really had any chance against Bucareli's forces.

BAUER ASSOCIATES, IMPORTERS

The monies authorized under Pidal's legislation were finally in Palma's hands by mid-August. It was a Tuesday when Emilia, Luis, Gregorio, and I drove in the Scout to Charlie Bauer's warehouse to search his catalogs.

Luis knew exactly the type of spray truck and equipment he wanted, and dutifully ordered fifty fully-equipped units.

"Luis my lad," Charlie told him, "you'd be running your pants off with fifty units in the field. You couldn't keep up with a tenth that many. That young son of yours would be saying, 'Momma, whose that bugger who runs in here on Sunday afternoon, eats an enchilada, and hightails it out of here Monday morning at first light?'"

"Order five this first time," Emilia suggested.

"Palma will not accept so small a number," Gregorio said. "His purpose is to create a enormously impressive show that will draw as much attention as possible."

I was intrigued by Gregorio's comment. It was the first indication I'd had as to whose camp he might be in.

"I agree," Luis said. "We must not take the chance of angering Palma. Perhaps half might be acceptable."

"Equipment changes so rapidly," Charlie said. "No use locking yourself into a truck model that is out-of-date the same year you buy it. He'll go for five; I'll fix it up with him. I'll tell him I talked you into five because I have inside information that they're coming out with something better next year."

Luis and Gregorio finally went along with that.

We applied the same basic philosophy to all our purchases that day. Larger orders could be made with more confidence after we'd tested the equipment.

In addition to the trucks, Luis had to buy backpack spray tanks; spare nozzles, hose, and other spare parts for the tanks; measuring and mixing containers; gloves, boots, and a hundred sundry items.

Charlie's skill was electrifying. Nothing was impossible. Trucks? Ten days at the most. *No problema.* Why should there be a problem. "I get cars—nearly any make—in less than a week out of Miami. Spray tanks? I can tell you in a matter of hours what they've got in stock." His huge bulk seemed everywhere as he thumped about, pulling catalog after catalog from his shelves and flipping almost to the page we sought as though he had them book-marked in some invisible way.

His detailed knowledge of the properties of all this stuff was also unbelievable. With Emilia's microscope purchases, his first question was, "Do you need oil immersion?" The average person wouldn't even think to ask.

"Yes, of course," Emilia said.

"Well, you said eggs. How am I supposed to know what kind of eggs? You could be talking fish eggs, in which case we could get by with a hand lens instead of a microscope. Let's get with it, Emilia; time is money."

It was interesting to watch Emilia work with him. His ribbing was obviously all in fun. She seemed to have rapport the others didn't, perhaps a friendship that had grown from frequent previous sessions of ordering.

She picked the laboratory tables for Corejo. These came with gas jets and the usual plumbing such as one sees in any school or medical laboratory. In addition to her microscopes, she ordered centrifuges, slides, coverslips, Canada balsam, formalin, acetic acid, stains, and a million other things.

Charlie could make a friend a minute with his expertise and efficiency. As I listened to his halting speech, and watched him move about his catalog sales office, it occurred to me that the frequent pauses in his sentences stemmed probably more from being out of breath than just from habit. It seemed likely that he had emphysema, although he didn't smoke, at least not in our presence.

In a way, I found myself feeling a bit sorry for this lonely man as I got to know him, living there alone amongst his catalogs, probably with few friends to socialize with in Aguilas. He appeared to have few outside interests. I learned that he didn't play golf, and he certainly wasn't built for tennis. He seemed nearly a prisoner in his own prison-like buildings. The windows were fitted on the outside with heavy iron bars. His daily contacts consisted mostly of haughty Aguilas upper-crust females accompanied by their chauffeurs, who came to select curtains for their dining rooms, lamps for their expensive tables.

However, he was not a morose individual in spite of his isolation. He helped us with boundless enthusiasm. Also, as I surmised from my first meeting with him on the plane, he managed some traveling. His entire mindset seemed constantly focused on his successful import business.

When it was my turn, Charlie seemed especially selective. Apparently, Palma had already discussed with him by telephone what I was entitled and not entitled to have.

"About this vehicle I'm supposed to order," was the way Charlie phrased it, "I can get you a delivery truck that will hold five men and all your equipment, but I don't want you out there on those back roads in something that isn't equipped to handle the places you'll be going. Those buggin' delivery trucks aren't built with strong enough springs and shocks for the game trails back up along the *Segre*."

A chill ran down my spine. Salvador and I had told no one except Emilia of our work at Hoof Print or the upper reaches of the *Segre*. I couldn't afford to risk losing the *Segre* to Luis's SCP. I prayed that Luis and Gregorio had not been listening closely enough to catch the drift of our conversation. Charlie knew exactly where Salvador and I had been working. He had to have learned it either from Emilia or from Marcos.

"And he specifically mentioned a delivery truck?" I asked.

"He was very clear about that," Gregorio said.

"We'll look like we're descending on a village to sell vacuum cleaners or magazine subscriptions. Should I order us identical uniforms?"

Charlie grinned, started to move on, but then came back to what I had just said. "Yes, with something appropriate embroidered on the shirt pockets. Or identical caps . . . visors . . . that's it . . . caps with visors. Harvey, Harvey! How have you managed to make yourself so unpopular? Have you been working at it, or does it come naturally? You're almost as bad as that Homma fellow you replaced. Good grief he was trouble!

"Of course, the sad part is that your crew will toast like muffins in any contraption built along the lines of a delivery truck. I'm thinking more of a used army truck, a World War II *six-by-six* with extra undercarriage an' plenty of traction. I can get you a six-by cheap."

"Sounds delightful," I said. "Nothing beats the patter of rain on a canvas roof, but I doubt Palma wants me to be that comfortable."

"Are there spare parts for a thing like that in case it breaks down?" Gregorio asked.

"*No problema!* There are parts scattered all over the globe. And I will explain to Palma that a six-by is guaranteed to bust the kidneys of the man in the passenger's seat in less than a month. He'll like that. You've really cooked your goose with him, Harvey. Shame on you. I thought you had more promise when we first met."

I couldn't imagine Palma confiding in Charlie about what a nuisance I had become. Maybe Emilia had described to him some of the high points of our staff meetings. Luis and Gregorio were watching me and enjoying Charlie's monologue. I'm sure I looked embarrassed.

Of course, I had boots, dip-nets, and containers to order, but my needs were minimal compared to Luis and Emilia. The only time Charlie seemed to draw a blank was when I asked for two more of Sam's filters so that I could keep two working and one in reserve. They weren't indexed anywhere, so he offered to have someone pick them up in San Juan if I could get Sam to provide them.

Something didn't quite ring true in the way Charlie insisted on the six-by. And he was pushing it in spite of the fact that he could make much more commission on a delivery truck. There was misfeasance there somewhere, but I didn't figure it out until much later.

We were through with our ordering long before quitting time, and we left Charlie copies of our preliminary lists in case we called in with changes after Gregorio cleared everything with Palma.

As we stepped out into the mid-afternoon sun. Emilia suggested we stop for coffee at Rubie's on the way back to the office. It was there that our conversation turned to Hernando's death, the hostility at Juncos, and what this sudden violence on the part of the soldiers meant both for *Terreno Difícil* and for the future of Tavira itself.

To my surprise, Gregorio seemed to be the most outspoken. We learned from him that Bucareli had already issued a fearsome order to the army: "no quarter; no prisoners." Gregorio felt that might have been behind the trigger-happy killing of Hernando. *Be first to draw blood,* sort of a macho reaction to such a grisly command. I was intrigued that Gregorio had information we had not heard, and that he chose to share it. Yet, apparently he was not party to the information about the shooters being members of Bucareli's personal guard. At least, he didn't let on if he were.

Luis was silent throughout this discussion. Hernando's death had probably depressed him since it came on his shift, and I'm sure my chiding of him that day was not forgotten. Most of the discussion was between Emilia and Gregorio. Emilia surprised me by revealing as much as she did about Marcos. Of course both Luis and Gregorio knew that Emilia and Marcos had been classmates in their youth. Hence, it seemed natural that she would have the inside track when it came to talking about Marcos's likes and dislikes, his morality, his idealism, things she might have remembered about him. However, Emilia went further than that, insisting that Marcos had the strength to drive Bucareli's army into the sea. She was feisty in her defense of him.

"Once he comes out of the *Espoleta*, the entire rural population will rally to him," she said.

"Great," Luis said, "Bolos battering Bucareli's tanks. Make quite a clamor." He picked up his coffee cup and pushed himself back ever so slightly from the table.

"You will see, Luis! I promise you," Emilia said. "Marcos has the capability of arming thousands of villagers."

Gregorio egged her on. "He will get thousands of villagers killed. That's about all he'll accomplish."

"Maybe they would rather die," Emilia said. "Maybe they would rather die free than live like they do; like their children must do after them, like their children's children must do after their children."

"Something like that," I quipped as we exchanged glances. Even as emotion played havoc with her sentence structure, Emilia's words were unmistakably *vintage Marcos.*

I knew it was for my benefit that all three of them had not lapsed into Spanish as they usually did when debating a hot issue over coffee at Rubie's.

I came away with the feeling that Gregorio was loyal to the Bucareli administration, but that they told him only what they wanted him to know.

It didn't surprise me that Luis confined his comments to schisto control and avoided politics completely. I had begun to understand that Luis was not a complicated man. Family, for him, as always, came first; job second; job politics third. I was learning that he was also a man of high integrity. A controlling sense of right and wrong pervaded everything he said and did.

THE DEPOT AT COREJO

My second or third-hand WWII army six-by-six was the first item on anyone's list to arrive at the wharf. Friday, September 4, Luis had one of his men drive it to the old leprosy sanatorium at Corejo.

Luis's five spray trucks arrived at the pier the following Monday, and stevedores offloaded twelve hundred pounds of SCP that came in on the same ship.

As soon as the items cleared customs, Luis and five of his newly hired drivers set off towards Corejo. I couldn't resist the opportunity to see how things were coming along. I was eager to have a look at my truck and to see where Luis had decided to park it.

Palma planned to assign the Scout to someone else as soon as I had the six-by ready for fieldwork. That meant that I would have to hook a ride from Aguilas to Corejo daily. That didn't present as much of a problem as I suspect Palma hoped it would. I soon found that I could ride with Luis or one of his men. I knew I would prefer that to driving the Scout alone all that way so frequently.

I had use of the Scout that Monday, however, and Emilia and I set off after Luis's convoy, arriving at the entrance gate to the leprosy compound in time to see Luis direct the parking of his five new trucks.

I was surprised at how emotionally disturbing it was for me to view the old barrack-style quarters at Corejo; rows of thin, plywood shelters that once housed hundreds of victims of a dread disease that for centuries turned mother, brother, sister, or friend into an instant outcast, never again to feel a comforting human hand or human hug.

It was an eerie feeling, and as I contemplated the life of those ghosts of Corejo, I recalled a moment eighteen years earlier when, while a venturesome youth, I was working one summer as a merchant seaman, and was climbing the dusty, unpaved road from the wharf at Buenaventura in Columbia. Of course today Buenaventura is a major seaport. Back then it was hardly more than a seaside village. As I ascended the hill, a leper approached, shuffling hurriedly towards me. Our eyes met as he passed. He held the lapel of his thin, black, robe-like garment pulled up to one side of his deformed face to protect himself from the village women as they screamed their curses and pelted him mercilessly with stones. The loneliness in his eyes has stayed with me ever since.

The facility at Corejo consisted of two sections: one for tuberculosis patients; the other, abandoned housing once occupied by hundreds of lepers. The barracks where the lepers had slept were arranged in a square that formed the border of a green area where huge gumbo-limbo trees shaded an undergrowth of hibiscus and bougainvillea. History has it that the Caribs, who were overrun and mostly murdered by the Conquistadors, used the resin from the gumbo-limbo trees as a poultice for bruises and sprains. I've always wondered if the lepers ever used it on their lesions. Perhaps that could explain such an unusual stand of gumbo in this strange and isolated seaside site.

The breeze off the ocean felt warm and clean. In the bright sunlight of that especially clear day, the aroma of seaweed and salt seemed almost therapeutic. No wonder the government had selected Corejo as the site for the TB sanitarium.

Emilia and I stood inside one of the old abandoned barracks, the one she planned to modify for laboratory use. It was light and well ventilated. However, I felt a curious presence as my eyes were drawn to first one and then another of the stark, rusting, iron cots that lined both sides of the room. No doubt, the straw mattresses had long since been burned. Better medicines had allowed the last few lepers to return home, sufficiently cured to live safely with their loved ones. Yet, the staff was reluctant to utilize the now vacant quarters, so great was their residual fear of the disease. Leprosy, a close relative of tuberculosis, has always received something of a bum rap. It always seemed strange to me that throughout history, and in vastly different parts of the globe, this least contagious disease of man should rouse almost irrational dread.

We joined Luis out behind the barracks in a huge lot where he planned to park his spray trucks. Of course, the five trucks on hand occupied practically no space at all. Still, they were an inviting sight, clean and new right down to their shiny hubcaps, and saddled with their bright white chemical tanks.

The twelve hundred pounds of SCP was stored in a supply barracks near the trucks. This barracks would hold Luis's replacement and reserve supplies as they arrived, and mine as well. My six-by had been assigned a premier parking spot next to the barracks door and beside where Luis's chauffeur had parked the company sedan.

Emilia didn't think much of my truck, and it was she who named it *Australorbis* to call attention to its snail-like get up and go.

Luis had hired special guards to man the gate and patrol the grounds. All Department of Health personnel had to have identification to enter. Luis had a considerable investment here in the compound and wasn't about to take the blame for theft or damage to his equipment.

Overall, that first day at Corejo was an exciting one. Seeing the extent of the new equipment, and imagining the day when ten times as many trucks would fill the parking lot, gave me a real feeling for the vast scope of Palma's project. I now had genuine reason to worry that I might not again find time to carry on my own protocol of field studies, that my time might be entirely consumed by Palma's extravaganza.

Towards four o'clock I decided to head back to Aguilas and turn in the Scout. Emilia rode with me. She seemed in a reflective mood.

"I do not expect the spraying to go smoothly," she said. "I do not think Marcos will sit still for it one minute. I fear there will be more shooting and more people killed as Marcos tries to make it too dangerous for Luis to get the work done."

"Who's he going to shoot? Certainly not the workers," I said. "He has a better sense of perspective than that."

"Soldiers! He will shoot the soldiers that Bucareli assigns to protect the spray teams."

"But they'd be sitting ducks. I don't see Marcos doing that. I know he hates the concept of spraying. Still, I see him finding some less savage route."

"Marcos can be tough as harness leather when he must be. But you are right. He hasn't the mindset of a true rebel."

"Is he just as he's always been? I mean, when you knew him back in high school? So many males seem to change completely when they get into a position of power."

"He never changed. Always the same. Then and now."

"But have you actually seen enough of him since 1953 to know he hasn't changed?"

"He has not changed. I know that."

"Do I detect more to your relationship with Marcos than meets the eye? I mean I see the way Luis and Gregorio seem always to defer to you whenever his name comes up in our conversations at Rubie's. It's as though they assign you the special role of speaking for him."

She didn't look at me. It was as if she didn't really want to answer. "Yes, they do. I . . ."

As she paused, I suddenly realized I was way out of bounds. I had no business quizzing her about a relationship that I sensed had a very personal side to it. I was trying to think how to reverse my invasion of her privacy when she said, "I should have told you sooner. I suppose, even though I trust you completely, I just did not see until now that it is vital you should know."

She was quiet for a long time before she said, "Marcos and I are married. We have been married since he came back in 1951. In fact, we were married at Juncos in Salvador's house. Salvador took a huge risk having the ceremony in his house. Salvador is like a father to Marcos. If Palma or Bucareli had ever found out, I hate to think what would have happened."

This news hit me like a sledgehammer. I'd begun to imagine that our relationship meant something more. I swallowed hard and tried to conceal the sense of contrition I felt for even thinking we could be more than friends.

"Why do you even still have your job?" I said. "They must know you two are married. Surely, your marriage certificate is on file. Why hasn't Bucareli told Palma to fire you long before this? Better yet, why hasn't he thought to play hardball, to use you to force Marcos to accept amnesty or something of that sort? Seems like Bucareli's wouldn't miss a bet like that."

"We were married informally, what you might call a common-law marriage," she said. "But more then that, it would be a weak bet. It would be the very worst bet Bucareli could make."

"Why do you say that?"

"Because if it did not work, and if it did not draw Marcos out, Bucareli would look the fool. Using a *woman*? He would most certainly expose himself to ridicule."

"But would it have worked?"

"Never. That is a decision Marcos and I agreed to as a shared vow at our marriage—no threat, no blackmail, even torture would not cause either of us to yield. Surely, Bucareli senses that. Bucareli fears Marcos because Marcos stands for candor and truth in an ethically impoverished land. The rural people trust Marcos. Those are the qualities that make Marcos dangerous to Bucareli. You do not get a man like Marcos to accept a compromise that would cause him to abandon a cardinal precept of his philosophy."

"So extortion is not an option Bucareli is likely to use?"

"Very *unsmart*!"

Corejo is farther north than Comerio. We had driven south from Corejo, turned east on the Juncos road, entered Comerio, and crossed the *Ebro* via the bridge in downtown Comerio. We were driving, now, along the bank of a narrow lowland creek set about with stilted huts. I knew it to be one of the streams Ota Homma had studied. At least a dozen children splashed about in the shallows, cooling off after a hot day perhaps in a hot schoolroom. I glanced at them quickly as we drove by. The road was too narrow and winding to allow me to pay much attention to their play. Yet, I had to say something to dispel the shock of Emilia's revelation.

"You have to wonder about their immunity," I said. "Certainly, they must develop considerable immunity spending as much time in the water as they do. You and I'd be dead in a year if we fooled around in water that dangerous."

Emilia's expression held a faint smile. I could sense that she felt their childish pleasure with the water. With her mother an attorney, her father a surgeon, there was no way she would ever have been allowed the freedom to swim in a river or stream. She grew up protected, chauffeured from school to piano lessons and to the country homes of school friends on weekends.

Marcos, too, had been an only child, except that his mother died in childbirth. Grandparents raised him. His father was a civil engineer in charge of the entire irrigation system for *Centrale Allende.* He'd earned a good salary. However, he was abruptly fired from his job in 1951 when Marcos, with his new law degree, returned from the States and tried to unseat Bucareli.

We drove on without saying anything more. She broke the silence as I turned in at the motor pool. "Come home with me and have dinner," she said. "We will have to improvise. I did not plan to invite you. I felt this morning that I might be quite fed up with you by the time we got back to Aguilas."

I laughed. "You sure know how to make a fellow feel welcome. All that silence, I thought I must *for certain* seem quite a bore."

She blushed.

After we left the Scout, reached the front of the building, crossed the street, and walked a few blocks west, she took my hand in hers and laced her fingers through mine as she had done at Hoof Print once before.

"You are not a bore, Harvey Shoals," she said. "Far from it. You have a busy mind that comes up with some bizarre but absolutely terribly smart ideas. And, of course, the fact that you never stop thinking in the abstract makes you quite safe to be with. How could we get into trouble when one of us cannot keep his mind on the tangible as opposed to the intangible for any significant length of time?"

"I'm sorry," I said.

"Well, that's okay. Marcos approves of you. I am permitted to spend all the time with you that I wish . . . with a few essential conditions, of course. Is that not a remarkable man, lonely as he is up there on the *Espoleta*?"

"He has a remarkable woman," I said. "Without your companionship and support, I probably would not have remained here this long. I considered pulling up stakes when Palma banned the overnight studies."

"*Pulling up stakes?* What do you mean?"

"I'm sorry again," I said. "Probably not quite the right connotation. Means *striking camp,* sort of like quitting or leaving."

"Watch Palma as this program unfolds," she said. "You will find that he will become as transparent as a jellyfish. He is almost as smart as some of them, too. Like some of the big dangerous ones with all the tentacles—like what you call . . . what is it in English? . . . the *Portuguese Man of War*.

"But he will not get away with his *Terreno Difícil*. Marcos will see to that. If Marcos does not stop him, Bucareli will. Maybe I kill him myself if I get a chance." Her black eyes flashed and as we walked she looked straight at me to see how I would react.

"I sense you don't care much for him," I said, expecting her to see the humor of my understatement.

"*Care for him!* Are you crazy?" she said. "I could never trust him enough to like him. I hate him. How could I like a man I cannot trust?"

When we entered her apartment, I noticed that the décor seemed much more feminine than the last time. She'd changed something. I couldn't identify exactly what. She fixed us both a margarita, encrusting the rims of both glasses with an especially heavy dose of salt. It had been a long hot day, and the salt hit the spot. Effortlessly, she threw together a tasty meal of shrimp scampi and homemade dinner rolls. We ate on our laps with the coffee table for our drinks. It seemed unlikely that she hadn't planned to invite me to dinner.

"You are kind," she said, "to say that my companionship helped you want to stay."

"Actually, it was more than that," I said. "In my own clumsy way, I fell hard for you, Emilia. I'm embarrassed to admit it, but it's true."

She studied me for a long time. "Your Maggie is dead, Harvey," she said quietly.

"Yes."

"Then that is why you let me think she is alive."

"*What* is why?" I asked. "What made you guess she's dead?"

"If Marcos were dead, do you think I would hesitate even one second before I could say *'I fell hard for you, too, Harvey?* I would practice it a hundred times until the chance to say it came. But in my heart Marcos will never be dead even if he is killed in the battle he seeks, and I would not say it if a thousand voices in my head screamed at me to say it. . . . Neither would you."

"I know," I said. I took her hands in both of mine.

Again, she laced her fingers between mine and then kissed me on the cheek. "Thank you, Harvey, for being a friend I can trust."

Later, as I rose to go, we stepped out onto her tiny deck to guess what kind of day the morning light might bring. The midnight air carried the scent of night-blooming jasmine and the shadows on the full moon stood out in high relief like great blue whales swimming the surface of a chromium sea.

THE CAMPAIGN TRAIL

With the arrival of the trucks and new equipment, a sense of urgency and optimism spread throughout the Department of Health. In the halls, Palma greeted section heads he hadn't encouraged for months, assigning them equipment and funds for every contingency.

From dawn to dusk, Luis and Emilia interviewed applicants for the new jobs. By the end of the week, Luis had five spray teams ready to begin work, Emilia had staffed the new lab at Corejo, and I'd picked the men I wanted to help me with the post-treatment surveys.

All of my five were from the Comerio area; all knew Salvador at least by name and reputation. Only my new driver, an older man by the name of Esteban Santiago, had a family to support. The other four were young, strong, and still single.

My crew, the six of us, took *Australorbis* for a test run to Valencia on Thursday, September 10. The engine had only sixty thousand miles on it, and the new canvas top reeked of fresh factory waterproofing. The test run wasn't intended for serious data collecting. I only wanted to judge the suitability of the truck when fully loaded and staffed, to acquaint my men with the equipment, and to give them a feel for the work we would be doing. It was a good day; the truck passed inspection; the men worked well together.

The following Tuesday, we did our first actual post-treatment survey as a team. I took them to Juncos. I'd been running hard to keep up with Luis at Juncos for nearly a month, and he planned to re-spray Wednesday afternoon. I had to get my survey done before he sprayed.

Unfortunately, we were rained out Tuesday before we finished. That meant returning Wednesday morning to finish the work, and of course that meant the platoon of guards would also need to return Wednesday morning. I told them we'd be along about mid-morning. Apparently, because of my short notice, Palma got confused, called the base, and ordered the platoon for 8 A.M.

We arrived about ten o'clock to find a platoon waiting. It was a different platoon and a different corporal in charge. They'd been waiting for three hours and the corporal was fighting mad.

"*El señor* Palma say you be here at eight! Why you not here on time?"

"I told yesterday's corporal we'd be here about mid-morning."

"Lieutenant tell us *el señor* Palma say 8 A.M."

I might have been more tactful if he hadn't been so belligerent. "You'll have to take that up with Palma," I said. "That's not my problem."

"We here to protect you. We need to know what time you get here!"

"Palma told you the wrong time." I started to say something disagreeable about "*el señor* Palma" but decided against it. After all, technically, this business of the riflemen was Bucareli's brainchild, not Palma's. "Even if we needed your protection, which we don't," I said, "Palma should realize there is no way I can get to Corejo, load my stuff, and drive to Juncos by eight o'clock. Even you should have brains enough to figure that out."

"So why he no say ten instead of eight?"

"Dammit! I already told you to take that up with Palma."

"We leave base at quarter to six. Much work to do."

"That's ridiculous!"

"Must scout perimeter; assign men to point; dig in."

"Look, Corporal, we don't need you. The villagers here are our friends. Just stay out of our way?"

"You need us if Marcos Díaz come."

"I need you least of all if Marcos Díaz comes."

He cursed and walked off to speak with his next in command.

For a while, the soldiers held to their assigned positions. However, as our work progressed, they gradually began to crowd around to see what we were doing. For the most part, the villagers stayed out of sight.

We were just finishing up when Luis and Palma arrived in Luis's chauffeured sedan, with one of the new spray trucks close behind. I guessed correctly that Palma came along to try a bit of campaigning. As he stepped out of the sedan, our corporal recognized him and called out an order that sent the platoon scurried to their assigned positions.

Luis's spray team shouldered their sprayers and trudged off up the hill to their starting point about five hundred feet upstream from where the vehicles were parked.

Palma walked over to the confluence of the *Perico* and the *Ebro*. He watched the river for a minute, and then he began walking upstream along the *Perico*.

I was eager to stay and watch Palma in action, and I asked Luis if I could ride back to Corejo in the sedan. Luis greeted that request with enthusiasm, apparently overjoyed to have someone along in the sedan in addition to Palma and the driver.

I dismissed my crew and told them to return to Corejo and take the rest of the day off.

Palma hovered over a couple of women washing clothes on the smooth stones at streamside. I heard him ask, "Is the water okay?"

One of them spoke. I couldn't hear her soft reply.

He said something in Spanish that sounded to me like, "My name is Harlan Palma, and my job is to be certain that the water here in your village is clean and safe for you to use."

The women said nothing.

He scratched around in the gravel at his feet, selected a flat stone the size of a fat silver dollar, and scaled it low over the water. It skipped on the water twice and landed in a stand of yellow allamanda thirty feet beyond the opposite bank.

I think he expected the two women to applaud. They didn't. The conversation went somewhat as follows.

"Do you have a son who can do that?" he asked them.

Neither answered.

"I learned to do that when I was a boy growing up in a village just like this one. My parents were cane-workers. We lived over close to Comerio."

I think he must have begun to sense hostility in the reaction of the two women. He glanced around. Luis and his men were several hundred feet upstream. They would start spraying just above the uppermost house. From that point, they would work their way downstream to the *Ebro*.

Palma turned to the women. "Okay, *señoras*. You can continue your washing just as soon we are finished."

"Why you want to spray here?" the oldest woman said. It was more a challenge than a question. She spoke loudly in English, perhaps so that Luis and I would hear.

"Spraying protects your health and cleans up the water," Palma said.

She said something about the soldiers and the guns; how they didn't want the guns.

Palma was quick to take advantage of the opportunity. "*Señoras*," he said, "I do not order the soldiers. President Bucareli orders the soldiers. He does not understand that you and Luis and I are friends. Luis and I have spent our lives working to bring better living conditions to the villagers in the *Espoleta*."

"Why they shoot Hernandos?" the woman asked.

"That was a terrible act," Palma said, "and I intend to see that the two soldiers responsible pay with their lives. All of the villagers of Juncos have my deep sympathy and Luis's deep sympathy."

Eventually, a group of workers came up the path from the direction of the *centrale*. Of course they all knew and respected Luis. His quiet deportment and sincere attitude, and the rural upbringing that had been his heritage, excused in large measure the harm spraying brought to the *Perico* and thus to all the villagers of Juncos The villagers had come to understand that Luis was only doing his job. Most of them had never met Palma and knew nothing about him. However, Marcelo, one of the younger men, recognized Palma and didn't hesitate to pick a fight.

"Have you come to watch the soldiers shoot our children!" he challenged.

"*Señor*," Palma said, "your village has the sympathy of all Tavirans. That *incident* was a tragic crime. The two soldiers responsible are presently charged with involuntary manslaughter. I will be watching the case closely to be certain that they are punished.

"*Incident!* Is that what you call it?"

I knew Marcelo to be a cousin to Hernando. I'd gotten to know and to like Marcelo months before when Salvador and I first started our work at Juncos.

Marcelo strode across the *Perico* to our side and approached Palma. "*Involuntary!* When a man points a gun and pulls the trigger, how can you say that is involuntary?"

"Their lawyer claims that they thought the youth was armed. They mistook him for a guerrilla. I think that is the general opinion of the government as well. However, if I were president, I would make it my duty to see that both are executed." Almost imperceptibly, Palma began to inch backward towards the sedan.

Marcelo followed, pushing closer, white knuckles gripping his machete. "Do we look like guerrillas? Do we look like big threat you have to shoot?"

I noticed that at least four members of the army squad had moved swiftly into position where they had a clear shot at Marcelo.

"I am as sorry as you that it happened," Palma said.

"It no happen if you no spray. We no ask you to do this to our *Quebrada Perico*."

"*Señor*," Palma said, standing his ground, no light between his pudgy belly and muscular Marcelo, "*el Perico* belongs to all of the people of Tavira. And Tavira wants its rivers and streams freed from the scourge of schisto."

I couldn't stay out of it. The situation was too dangerous. Palma's approach was not right, and Marcelo's machete was only inches from his face.

I knew Marcelo was no fool, but at that moment, his machete seemed far sharper than his mind.

Marcelo," I said, "out of respect for Salvador . . . stop now before there is more shooting."

Another man in the group put a gentle hand on Marcelo's shoulder and spoke softly, "*Sí. Marcelo. Vámonos!* Fault not *el señor* Palma. He work for *el señor* Bucareli just as we do."

After a long, tense moment, Marcelo's machete arm relaxed, and the weapon dangled at his side. He grinned at me as he backed away. I think he was glad for a way out.

Palma cast me a bewildered but somewhat grateful look. The crisis was over, and he had planted a couple of seeds that could easily begin to take root if carefully nourished in the weeks ahead. On balance, both with the two women and then the men, I think he won some votes that day.

BUSHWHACKED

AT VALENCIA

There were several other times during September when Palma joined Luis in the field in a brave effort to win the vote of the villagers. He handled himself well, using every opportunity to shift the blame to Bucareli for sending the soldiers, promising to keep the pressure on to see that Hernando's killers paid with their lives. Clearly, Bucareli's efforts to discredit him had backfired. Palma was indeed a resourceful opponent.

Luis was now spraying the *Segre* as well as the *Perico* and a dozen other streams in the *Espoleta*. Palma often accompanied him, and Luis would dutifully report Palma's vote-getting encounters to me or to Emilia, even to Gregorio, often over coffee at Rubie's. It soon became obvious to us that Palma's grand strategy in the contest for the presidency could indeed succeed. Towards the end of September, he was actually attracting a gathering of villagers each time he went along. He had formulated a strong platform: First, he would allege that he had the expertise to rid their valley of disease, and as president he would have access to the funds with which to do it. Second, he would imply that Bucareli's factory was robbing them blind, that if he were president they would never again be in debt to the store at *la centrale*.

Monday, October 5, my men and I had been working at Valencia in advance of Luis's spray team, which was due to arrive towards afternoon. The platoon of soldiers that had accompanied us had orders to remain at Valencia while Luis's sprayers did their work.

Things had been quiet—exceptionally quiet. Few villagers were out and about—exceptionally few. I assumed the village women were busy with housework, if there were housework to do in those tiny dwellings. From the outset, I sensed a foreboding that I couldn't identify.

My men were packing *Australorbis* to leave when the spray truck arrived. Seconds later, Luis and Palma drove up in the chauffeured sedan.

As Luis's men adjusted the straps on their backpack sprayers, donned their spray masks, and set off upstream along the dirt and gravel road that followed the bank of the *Segre*, I asked Luis if I could again hook a ride back with him. As I expected, he welcomed the suggestion.

I told my men to finish packing up and to return to Corejo, again giving them the rest of the day off.

Palma had walked down to the bank of the *Ebro*, and was casually studying the acres of sugar cane across the river that stretched as far as the eye could see. There were no villagers about for him to lobby. He soon returned to talk to Luis. Occasionally, I'd see a woman scurrying along the spider-web of trails that joined one stilted hut to the next.

Suddenly, all five of Luis's spray team came trotting back down the hill from the way they'd gone. They were jabbering so rapidly and excitedly that I could decipher less than half of what they said. Apparently, they'd seen something over on a low ridge to the northeast, perhaps the same thing that had the village women ill at ease.

One of the soldiers fired a shot. I looked quickly. His weapon was pointed northeast. Another soldier fired. Soon the entire squad was expending round after round, firing at what to me was an unseen enemy. Their corporal was running around in circles giving orders. He called to Luis at one point. I realized that he was ordering Luis to pack up on the double and leave so that he and his soldiers could leave. Apparently, he sensed from what the spray team had said, that he was badly outnumbered.

Abruptly, shadowy figures emerged from the woods along the top of the low ridge. They were dressed in fatigues, wore no helmets, and appeared armed only with rifles. The platoon continued firing and the men on the ridge returned fire. Several rounds hit the spray truck.

A round pierced the backpack sprayer worn by one of Luis's crew, and the man froze in an expression of comical bewilderment as a shower of pressurized, concentrated SCP soaked him from head to foot. The corporal got him in the protection of one of the trucks and doused him with the last of their drinking water. Luis called to the corporal to order the man strip and dive in the *Ebro*. The concentrated SCP would have burned his skin and could have produced a dangerous and persistent inflammation. The muddy *Ebro* presented far less risk.

I'd been studying the ridgeline. When I next looked around, Luis and Palma were standing close to one another fifty feet from the sedan. Neither moved. They presented a perfect target. I was about to call to them to take cover, but, at that instant, a burst of gunfire came from the ridge, and Palma staggered backward and fell; Luis was not hit. I ran to them and Luis and I lifted Palma—Luis the arms, I the legs—and carried him to the sedan where we laid him carefully on the gravel. I folded a soft pillow from the sedan and put it under his head, realizing as I did so that it was pointless. From the looks of it, Palma had been hit in the chest by several rounds. There was no pulse. He had died almost instantly.

"We need to get him to better cover than this," Luis said. "Let me send my crew on their way, then I'll come back and help you move him."

"He's gone," I said. "There's nothing we can do for him. We'd best take cover till this is over."

"I knew it!" Luis said. "I knew the instant I heard the bullets thump into Palma's chest that several of them must have aimed and fired on command. That's when I knew I was not in harm's way. They wanted Palma. Marcos wanted Palma dead. What a blunder! He has written his own death warrant this time."

By now, the corporal and his squad were dug in behind driftwood and still firing at the ridge. I soon noticed that there was no return fire. Whatever the force up there, they'd given no indication that they intended to advance. I peered cautiously around the front of the sedan. I saw no one on the ridge. I turned to catch the corporal's attention and mimed an exaggerated shrug. Quite obviously, it was over.

Eventually, the corporal ordered his men to pack up their equipment and be ready to move out. Luis decided that we should take Palma's body to the hospital at Comerio. Four soldiers loaded the body across the back seat of the sedan.

Significantly, no one other than Palma had been hit and the spray truck was only slightly damaged. A tire on the north side was shot out and there were bullet holes in the door. Luis's men appeared badly shaken. As two of them changed the tire, they told me they'd spotted the aggressors on the ridge as they walked up the gravel road beside the *Segre*.

Luis ordered his chauffeur to ride back to Corejo on the spray truck so Luis and I could have both front seats.

As we prepared to follow the spray truck towards Allende Bridge, Luis repeated his assertion. "He wanted Palma. He's doomed now for certain."

"I'm not so sure it was Marcos," I said. "I think Marcos would have attacked from due north, possibly coming down the road directly behind your retreating sprayers. He'd have wanted to make his escape to the north. You can't escape to the north from that ridge. The escarpment is in the way. The ridge is between the road and the escarpment."

"Are you certain?"

"I'll show you what I mean on the way out. This wasn't Marcos's work. I'll bet you a Coca Cola it was Bucareli's shooters!"

We had only to drive a few hundred yards to prove my point. The ridge lay south of the escarpment in plain view from the road. "Marcos would never risk picking a spot where chance could trap him between two hostile forces. Do you want to look around in there for tire tracks? It wouldn't take but a minute."

"God no!" Luis said, laying a heavy foot on the gas pedal. They could still be there."

"Just kidding," I said. "Sorry. Thought I might get a laugh out of you."

He took his eyes off the road just long enough to glance at me. Then he turned back to face the road. Perhaps it was my imagination, but I thought I detected a faint trace of a smile. "You are a regular *pistol*, Harvey," he said, "and you can take that as a compliment."

As we drove along in the dust-cloud behind the spray truck, I asked how he thought we ought to report what had happened. I figured we ought to be together as to what we had observed.

"We'll drop Palma off at the hospital morgue," he said. "We need to contact Bucareli's office, preferably before the corporal can get to a telephone. I will make the call from the hospital and I will say as little as possible."

At the hospital, several workers helped to transfer Palma's body to a gurney. A physician counted five chest wounds. I gave them a brief account of the battle while Luis called Bucareli's office. Then we left them and headed for Corejo.

"Do you think Bucareli could order a killing like that and be able to find a half dozen men he could trust to carry it out and keep the secret?" I asked.

"He could find a hundred," Luis said. "Like all evil leaders, he could find a hundred."

So Luis had no trouble accepting my theory. I knew Emilia would agree. This was not Marcos's style.

When we reached Corejo, Luis checked on his spray team and signed off on the return of the truck. We counted exactly five bullet holes in the passenger side of the door. Except for the tire, there was no other damage. It was almost as if the leader of Bucareli's little force had told his men to each put a round through the truck door, but to avoid hitting any of the soldiers. They'd come with a mission to accomplish. They'd carried it out successfully.

From Corejo to Aguilas, Luis and I speculated on whom Bucareli would appoint to run the Department of Health, and what the new man's policies might be.

As I write this, I'm surprised I didn't think to cable George Barlow at the PDS that very evening and explain that things were falling apart on Tavira. I should have asked to be withdrawn immediately. If I'd acted promptly, the situation for me might not have gotten out of hand.

THE NEW DEAL

Bucareli was in Palma's office the following morning when I arrived at the Department of Health. The receptionist called to me as I entered the building. "Doctor Shoals," she said, her English a halting but emotionless monotone, "Doctor Palma is dead. Guerrillas . . . yesterday . . . at Valencia."

"Yes, I was there," I said, "but don't jump to conclusions." I realized as I said it that it was a dumb thing to say.

She looked at me for a moment, her mouth slightly open, dark eyes staring. Then, abruptly, she snapped her mouth shut and swallowed. "They want you upstairs in Doctor Palma's office."

I thanked her and punched the elevator button.

Upstairs in the hall, Emilia grabbed my sleeve with both hands. She was just emerging from the lavatory.

"Are they out of paper towels?" I quipped, feeling of her moist hands.

She slapped at me playfully, then grimaced, nodding towards Palma's office. "It's Bucareli himself in there! Please be careful. If he were to—"

"He won't," I said.

"Charlie warned me yesterday this would happen. He wanted me to know *in advance* that Marcos was not involved."

"Well, don't breath a word about *that*," I said. "There's enough trouble in that tip-off to get Charlie killed, too." She was obviously frightened and expecting the worst by the time we reached the door to Palma's office.

"May I pretend that you and I are kind of close?" she asked. "It could help to maintain my cover."

I couldn't help being amused. She hadn't done a lot of worrying about her cover up till now. Apparently, she genuinely feared Bucareli.

As we entered the room, I said to her quietly, "My love, you run a fine laboratory. I've always been especially attracted to laboratory technicians."

"Really?"

"Absolutely. As a group, they tend to be highly egocentric, their interests and conversation rarely transcending the bounds of their job description."

"Gotcha!" she said, smiling for the first time.

Bucareli displayed boundless energy. He was all over the room, greeting people as they came in, hugging women of all ages, sizes, and shapes, and vigorously backslapping male subordinates and supporters alike. He was far more gregarious than I expected; hardly the aloof, disturbed, textbook totalitarian that I'd rather assumed he would be. He was heavy-set, tall, with plenty of muscle under the short sleeves of his nylon, imitation rice-shirt. As the owner of *Centrale Allende* and president of Tavira, his influence, even without his bodyguards and private army, was obviously impressive.

He moved through the crowd with assurance. He noticed immediately Emilia's apparent interest in me as we stood close to each other near the window in the alcove of Palma's office. "Aha," he said. "So you two have found each other?"

It seemed a casual test to see how we would reply. I assumed from the way he'd worded his question that he at least knew *something* about me.

"So you know Emilia?" I said.

Emilia blushed and said nothing.

"One of the most rewarding aspects of my work," I said, "is getting to know so many of the people in each location who have devoted their careers to working on the schisto problem."

"Yes," he said, somewhat indifferently. "I imagine so. And we must always remember that teamwork is king," adding, "A lot of the think-tankers that have come steaming in and out of Aguilas over the last decade failed to deliver a dime's worth of value in exchange for the funds spent to send them here. Glad you are someone we can talk to and learn from." Then, he finally got to the questions that I knew must be on his mind. "So you saw Harlan killed?"

"Yes. He died almost instantly."

"Did it look to you as though he were a target? In addition to the truck, I mean. Or even *the* target, perhaps?"

So he'd gotten a detailed report. Before I could answer, Charlie Bauer pushed his way between us and picked up on Bucareli's question, "No doubt about it. He was *the* target. Five rounds to the chest, no one else even scratched? There's no contesting that. Irrefutable, I'd say."

I was surprised that Charlie butted in, and I wondered where he'd gotten the accurate figure of "five rounds to the chest." I wondered if he'd intervened primarily to take the heat off Emilia, or just to stay abreast of what we might say.

Bucareli spoke next. "Well, we have all worried about him. He has been a brave soldier in this fight against snail fever for a long, long time. He is a national hero. We owe him a great debt. One thing you can be certain of: Marcos Díaz will pay dearly for this dastardly unprovoked attack. Retribution will be forthcoming! And soon!"

And so the meeting went.

After about forty-five minutes of pretense like that, Bucareli stepped briefly to a podium they'd set up, and asked for quiet. His eulogy for Palma was the essence of what he'd just said to Emilia, Charlie, and me. I couldn't seem to muster any emotion regarding Palma's death. My heart ached instead for Salvador. Bucareli killed Hernando for the same reason he'd killed Palma: solely to ensure his success in an election.

Before Bucareli finished speaking, he pronounced Gregorio head of the Department of Health. That was it. The meeting broke up. No two people could have been more surprised than Emilia and I. Neither of us had the slightest hint as to what the appointment meant nor where it would lead. I think Emilia was stunned. I know she had expected and hoped for an outsider who might be open to other ways of controlling schisto than by the unwholesome use of environmentally destructive chemicals such as SCP.

We had few clues as to the direction Gregorio might go. None of us knew his true feelings regarding the use of SCP. He had not once, in Palma's presence or at Rubie's, commented regarding SCP, or discussed any of my field studies as they might relate to developing an environmentally safe control program. He'd conversed freely at Rubie's about many other things, but he'd left those subjects alone.

FLIGHT OF THE CONDOR

Before Palma's assassination, the days seemed to race past in weeklong blocks rather than one at a time. Luis was working a dozen streams, and I'd hardly finish one follow-up study before I'd have to go somewhere else and start another. That left my own research, the cercarial and snail studies, at a standstill.

However, after Palma's assassination, Luis, on orders from Gregorio, quit spraying. We were thrown into a state of limbo while the government assessed the situation. I had the strong feeling that Gregorio was receiving orders from Bucareli and did not have a free hand to direct Department of Health policy.

By late-October I'd pretty much caught up with Luis. In fact, I'd had time to assemble a substantial manuscript that I entitled "Snail Repopulation Following the Chemical Treatment of Streams." The data confirmed Salvador's and my suspicions that as snails returned, cercarial levels in the water actually rose to much higher levels than before SCP was applied to the stream. This unfavorable result, I attributed to two factors: 1. The killing of guppies through application of the chemical. 2. The fact that infected snails, due to their impaired ability to cling to vegetation, tended to be washed downstream from upland tributaries more easily than their healthier siblings. This second explanation was largely speculation, but I thought it worth suggesting.

I also had time to put my crew to work learning the rudiments of conducting basic rather than applied research.

My usual day began in Aguilas early each morning as I waited outside the hotel for my ride to Corejo. I usually got to Corejo about eight o'clock. My crew would drift in somewhere around nine.

Thursday, October 29, when I arrived at Corejo, I walked from the entrance gate towards my cramped office. I had to walk that short distance because the fellow who brought me from Aguilas to Corejo that day worked over at the TB sanatorium some distance from the gate.

As I rounded a corner of our barracks I noticed a small figure climbing out of the opening in the canvas at the back of *Australorbis*. I stopped in my tracks just as the individual looked up. I realized it was Salvador!

"*Great Scott* but you gave me a start," I called out to him. "How did you get past the guards?"

"*No problema, doctor*, they know me. Anyway, I tell them I drive for you today. Esteban Santiago not come to work today."

"You may drive if you wish," I said, smiling as I added, "Salvador, this is wonderful. I'm so happy to see you!"

His magnificent smile was missing. I hoped that his grief had not stolen that away from him forever. We talked for a few minutes beside the truck. I could see that he'd been inside the barracks because the door was open and the ceiling light was on. Esteban must have loaned him his keys.

There was a box on the ground between us. Salvador picked it up and lifted it into *Australorbis*. I realized that it was a box of SCP from Luis's half-ton supply. "Why are you loading that?" I asked.

"*El señor* Luis ask me to bring it. I think he store all SCP at *la centrale*. Maybe more easy if he keep it there."

"You mean all of it?"

"*Sí.*"

The idea struck me as incredulous, but *Australorbis* was the only vehicle with room for moving a half-ton of anything. The spray trucks hardly had a square inch of storage space once loaded for the field.

I asked him about his new job up at Marcos's encampment. He explained that Marcos had put him in charge of supply which I already knew, and that the work kept him running from one end of the *Espoleta* to the other.

"You know, *doctor*, we right. Marcos get message from *el señor* Bauer when supply ship come. Men go to north beach to unload. I tell Marcos what come. Then Marcos say what to bring south and what store in caves in north."

I was surprised that he kept no secrets from me. "What kind of shape are his guerrillas in?" I asked.

"Very strong, *doctor*. They will win. When day comes, they win."

"How can you be sure?"

"You must believe. If you see his supplies, you believe."

My men had begun to appear. Salvador and I dropped the subject quickly. His information was too sensitive to risk having it overheard. By nine-thirty we were loaded and ready to go. With Salvador driving, we were fully staffed. None of the men seemed surprised to see Salvador. They all greeted him warmly. As I watched him with the others, I realized that he was not himself. He had lost a lot of weight and aged terribly since Hernando's death.

As we headed for Valencia, he asked, "*Doctor*, you finish work at Hoof Print?"

"Yes. And I would have done more downstream in the *Perico* if I'd had you to help me."

"You are kind, *doctor*. I am sorry. But there is not much time. When Marcos win, then you fix schisto the right way, not wrong way. First Marcos, then schisto."

"How is your daughter, Francesca . . . is that right? Yes. How is Francesca managing without Hernando?" I asked.

"She cook at Marcos camp now. Everyone in Juncos who not work for *la centrale* work for Marcos."

"I'm sorry, Salvador. I've kicked myself a thousand times for not trying harder to make Palma understand that our work did not need soldiers. I never even dreamed they'd shoot a villager."

"No your fault. Men who kill Hernando work for Bucareli. They kill Hernando on purpose."

I didn't need to quiz him further because I realized that he had been way ahead of me all along. Yet, if his hatred for the government prevented him from working with me any longer in spite of how much he enjoyed the work, why was he filling in for Esteban Santiago today? I changed the subject.

We talked of many things on the way to Valencia. I mentioned his weight loss. It was terribly noticeable as he sat at the wheel, his skinny legs like pipe-stems reaching to the pedals through tattered fatigues. Purple veins tracked in high relief over the wasted muscles of his forearms. He did not look at all well.

I asked when had he last seen a physician. How was his appetite? Had he any unusual aches or pains? He shrugged off my questions.

"*Doctor*, you know what happen?" he said. "When I young *machetero*, cutting cane all day, I get stronger each day—so strong I think maybe I can lift up front of this truck. I lift front of Volkswagen in Comerio one time."

"You're putting me on."

"*No, doctor*. This is true. I pick up front so *mi sobrino* can put piece of wood under car and work under car."

"Maybe you imagined you did that. Maybe he picked it up and you put the wood under the frame."

"I lift it, *doctor!* . . . Now, I work but I get weak, not strong."

He stopped talking to negotiate the traffic at the Allende Bridge. Salvador had never improved at being able to talk in English while driving in traffic at the same time.

La Zafra, the harvest, was in full swing. However, tomorrow was a holiday, Tavira's special Columbus Day, the day on which Columbus, on one trip or another, was said to have visited Tavira.

"What a lot of activity," I commented.

"*La centrale* close *mediodía.*"

"At noon. Yes," I said."

At the north side of the bridge, I was surprised that Salvador turned left towards Valencia instead of going first to drop the SCP off for storage at the *centrale*.

"But you work with head," he said. "Do you think it is same? Your brain grow tired when you are eighty?"

"Excuse me," I interrupted, "aren't you supposed to take the SCP to *la centrale*?"

"We do that on way home," he said offhandedly. "Do you think brain grow tired like body?"

"Your brain hasn't," I said, glad to be out of the crush of traffic on the bridge, and aware that his questions were intended to distract my concern for the SCP. "I guess it makes you feel pretty good to be working for Marcos," I added.

"*Sí*. Maybe when Francesca's María have children, maybe María say to them, 'Your great-grandfather fight with Marcos Díaz. Your great-grandfather fight with Marcos Díaz when the armies of *el señor* Juan Bucareli fight guerrillas at battle of Valencia!'"

There was something wistful in his tone, I looked at him and said quietly, "Yes . . . maybe they will say something like that."

He kept his eyes on the road, and in a way, he seemed to be purposely avoiding looking my way. Then, quickly, and for only a moment, he turned his head towards me, the lines of his weather-beaten face tracing out a bittersweet grin that seemed to accent the emaciation so evident in the rest of his frame. But he didn't speak.

When we parked at Valencia, he was the first out and full of commands for the four men in back. Curiously, the usual squad of soldiers had not arrived. Possibly they got a late start from Comerio, but more likely, Bucareli had retracted that ridiculous order now that Palma was dead.

My crew moved north along the edge of the *Segre*. Salvador didn't accompany them, but they paid attention to the barrage of orders that he called after them in Spanish. I couldn't make out half of what he told them. But I could see that he held their respect. It was a pleasure to see that. He deserved it.

Surprisingly, Luis arrived in his sedan with Emilia. His chauffeur was not with him. His crew had the day off and he was not there to spray. Emilia promptly headed upstream following my crew. She didn't stop to chat, although I rather hoped she would. Salvador had gone over to *Australorbis* and was wiping down the windshield.

I casually mentioned to Luis that I had the half-ton of SCP in the back of the truck.

"You have what?" he said. He sounded tired, but our eyes met as he tried to sort out that revelation. He seemed distraught over something, but it certainly wasn't the SCP.

"I didn't load it, Salvador did," I said, wanting to test him on this matter a bit further.

"When?" still somewhat indifferently.

"He was loading it when I got to Corejo this morning. He had one box yet to put on the truck. I asked him what the deal was. He said you have decided to store it at *Centrale Allende*."

Gradually, the wheels began turning in Luis's mind. He didn't take his eyes off me. I expected him to turn and call out to Salvador to come and explain things. He didn't. Instead, he said quietly but firmly, "My guess is that you have about one minute to decide where you want to spend the next few weeks. Whether you noticed it or not, your men have already begun moving north into the woods, and Emilia is with them."

"She always does that. She wants to talk to Marcos."

"Well, this time, if my guess is correct, she won't be coming back."

"What do you mean?"

He looked around quickly. "Harvey, I have a family to attend to. There's no time. I am heading back right this second. Come with me. This is not your fight or mine." With that, he got back into the driver's seat of his sedan and started the engine.

Ten seconds later a dozen mortar rounds streaked overhead, exploding high up in the watershed. Luis signaled me with his hand to get in the sedan. I started to open the door, but looked around when I heard the truck engine start and saw Salvador behind the wheel. Salvador gunned *Australorbis's* engine and aimed the big chassis uphill.

I glanced back at the *Ebro*. The shallow river was alive with soldiers, hundreds of them wading across the current towards our shore. In the distance, along the road from Allende Bridge, I could hear the ominous approach of tanks. The clank and screech of their massive treads was punctuated by the explosion of mortar rounds which streamed overhead in ever larger volleys.

I waved Luis off and slammed the sedan door, but I did not intend to just stand there in the midst of a battlefield. I ran to catch *Australorbis*. As I struggled to open the door and pull myself into the passenger seat beside Salvador, I shouted, "Where in Sam Hill do you think you're going?"

"Go back with *el señor Luis, doctor*. You will be safe."

"Did you know this would happen today?"

"*Sí, doctor!*"

"How?"

"*El señor* Bauer tell Marcos."

"And Emilia?"

"Maybe too Emilia."

I thought of jumping out. I knew Salvador couldn't risk stopping to let me out. If he did, he'd be overrun by the foot soldiers who were now running towards us and rapidly closing the gap. My curiosity was aroused. I wanted more answers.

"Did Luis know this would happen today?"

"No. But he figure it out." He turned to grin at me for the second time all day.

"When did Marcos know?"

"*Anoche*. Last night."

So they *did* have some sort of radio contact, Charlie and Marcos.

Salvador now had *Australorbis* climbing the hill faster than the soldiers could run. We passed two of my crew who were obviously winded. Salvador chose not to stop and pick them up but called to them to grab hold behind.

"How did my men know they were supposed to move north into the woods? When did they learn of this?"

"*Anoche*," he repeated.

"From whom?"

"Marcos have many messenger."

It began to come clear to me. That explained why Esteban was missing. Like Luis, he was a family man.

It was soon obvious that Bucareli's force was much stronger than Marcos had expected. Marcos's forward scouts had been in amongst the houses not far upstream when we arrived. We passed several of them hurrying up the gravel road. Tanks were advancing rapidly now behind us. I could hear the roar of their diesel engines as the treads slipped and ground on the smooth gravel of the *Segre*. No doubt, the foot soldiers had fallen in behind the tank column.

Salvador swung *Australorbis* east on the branch road that lead toward Hoof Print. I caught a glimpse of Marcos, pistol in hand, Emilia at his side. What a pair they made! They were together at last. I don't think they saw me in the front seat next to Marcos, and I had no way of knowing then that this was to be the last time I would see either of them for many years to come.

I asked Salvador why he was heading east.

"They are too close."

"Dammit, Salvador, that's not an answer! They'll chase us down. There's no way out from this road. You know that as well as I do!"

Salvador was too preoccupied to answer. "We stop *momentito*. Then you get out."

Ahead I noticed a shabby group of guerrillas waiting at the side of the road. They had a huge pile of what looked like old quilts lying by the side of the road. Salvador stopped *Australorbis* beside them, leaned out the window, and spoke quickly. Next came the thump of feet as several men entered the back of the truck. Near silence followed. They were loading something aboard—speaking quietly amongst themselves.

In moments, the loading was done. The men jumped out and ducked into the forest. Salvador gunned the engine. I guess he realized that he didn't have time to argue with me there. Soldiers were close behind us on the road and firing into the trees in the direction of the fleeing guerrillas. They'd probably have shot me as I left the truck.

What Salvador had in mind didn't occur to me until we actually reached the fork where the side road curved south, downhill towards Allende Cliff. Salvador applied the brakes at that junction after turning the front wheels slightly to the right.

"Okay, *doctor*, now I go alone."

"You mustn't do this Salvador. It's too dangerous."

"*Por favor, doctor* . . . go!" he ordered softly.

I didn't budge. In my side mirror I could see the soldiers again. I said, "Move it, Salvador. The soldiers are closing in."

He gunned the engine and *Australorbis* began to roll downhill.

"Okay," I said, "as soon as you put distance between us and the soldiers, get her going straight. Then both of us will jump free and make for the woods."

"No good," he said. "Must keep wheels straight."

It was then that I guessed the wider purpose of Salvador's plan.

"What did they load back there?" I asked quietly. I'd already guessed.

"Nitro."

It figured. Nitro, carefully padded, plus a half-ton of very unstable SCP, and hot boilers down below, perhaps even overheated from working from dawn until noon. It would make quite a pyrotechnic display. Obviously, this stunt had been arranged carefully long before Marcos knew of the impending attack. I'd stepped into the middle of a nightmare, and Salvador was getting awfully nervous because of my presence.

"Please, *doctor*. You must jump. Soldiers stop at top of hill. Jump. Run east to Juncos. They help you at Juncos!"

"You mustn't do this," I said. You have friends, *amigos*, down there *en la centrale*."

"*La centrale* close *mediodía*." Then, turning towards me, he laughed. "I *hope* they close *mediodía*."

He was enjoying this! He floored the accelerator for a brief moment. The heavy truck bounded downhill toward the edge of the escarpment.

I kicked my door wide open. "I want to see you open your door right this second," I said. "I want to see you ready to jump."

Obligingly, he pulled on the door handle and kicked his door open on its rusty hinges. With wings outstretched and the wind whistling through the cab, the old truck looked like some sort of giant condor as it raced towards the edge of the escarpment. The jarring was intense except in those moments when we seemed nearly airborne.

"Now!" he commanded.

I faced him. Tears glistened in his eyes. Then he called, "We jump!"

He cast me one final comforting Salvadorian grin. I gave him a parting punch on the right shoulder, turned, and pushed off, hoping against hope to avoid a concussion and a bunch of broken bones.

As I hit the ground, I recall hearing the pounding tires as the primitive rocky road continued to punish *Australorbis* in her race towards the escarpment. There was a moment of silence, maybe three seconds. Then the rocks beneath my body heaved with the violence of an explosion such as I never hope to hear again, and a column of black smoke and debris, wide as a city block, rose silently hundreds of feet above the escarpment.

Seconds later, stones, hot coals, bits of cement, plaster, and wood, followed by a steaming, smelly shower of boiling sugar cane, pummeled me as I lay there cut and bruised, both my hands clutching at shrubs. I'd landed less than thirty feet from the rim of the escarpment, sliding as I struck the ground.

I was coughing. The sharp rocks and falling debris had cut and seared me badly in a hundred places. I looked around enough to see that I was safely away from the edge, and I sat up quickly.

"Salvador!" I called.

Desperate as I knew our situation to be, I was in a mood to tease him a bit about his driving.

There was no answer.

I rose to my feet and looked carefully around. He was nowhere. I limped to the edge of the escarpment. *Centrale Allende* was decimated, the smokestack completely gone. The huge boilers had burst, sending shrapnel crashing through the walls in a hundred places, collapsing all but the north wall which now leaned imperfectly against the cliff.

I backed away. Shots fired from up the hill brought me to my senses. Searing flames reached nearly to where I stood, igniting shrubs along the edge of the cliff only a few yards away. Smoke filled the sky. Already, a faint breeze from the west had carried a great wide swath of smoke at least as far as Juncos.

Surely, they knew in Juncos what the blast and smoke meant, and I had little doubt they also knew that Salvador was dead.

Escape

Six soldiers had fanned out on the road above me, heading down towards me. I had two obvious options: I could surrender or try to escape to the east. I chose the latter and ran limping and stumbling east along the crest of the escarpment. Several rounds of rifle fire narrowly missed me just as I dove into dense forest.

If I can just keep ahead of them, I told myself, *and if they don't strike a course to cut me off, they'll soon tire of the game and head back to their unit.* My cuts and burns were hurting, and I was out of breath, but I had to keep pushing on to the east until I intercepted a tributary of the *Perico.* Just one tributary, no matter how small, was all I needed. I would follow it down to Juncos.

I'd gone about a mile when, suddenly, my shoes felt heavy as cast iron, like one of those terrible nightmares of trying to run but too tired to lift one's feet. It took me a moment to gather my senses and realize that my shoes had filled with water. I slipped on a submerged stone and sat down hard in the middle of a stream. I rose, limped through the shallow water to the east bank, and turned to follow it south toward the village.

I passed two shanties and several villagers before I realized what an apparition I must present, clods of debris from the explosion caked to my clothes by a tenacious paste of drying molasses.

The news of my presence preceded me throughout the watershed. I was still following just a tributary and not the main stream when someone called to me. "*Doctor*, come quickly! This way." It was Francesca. She hustled me into a sort of utility space attached to her home and ordered me to strip. Averting her eyes, she returned with a pot of hot water, soap, and a towel. Finally, she laid out some of Hernando's college clothes, including his college cap, sweatshirt, and pants. It was an effective disguise.

On the mountain, I had protected my face from the falling debris, but the rest of my body was severely cut and bruised. The hot water burned but was comforting.

That evening, Francesca called a meeting of several villagers to discuss what should be done with me. I listened over a cup of strong coffee. Their decision seemed logical. They would send me off on the school bus in the morning after swearing the school children to silence. Felipe, the driver, could be trusted. After dropping the kids at their school in Comerio, Felipe would seek to determine if the authorities were looking for me. Based on what he learned, he would tell me what I should do next. If they were after me, Francesca had cousins in Comerio who could hide me for several days at least.

The meeting broke up as soon as those decisions were reached. No one seemed in a mood to ask questions.

Only Marcelo questioned me briefly. "Did Salvador jump free," he asked.

"No," I had to tell him.

Salvador had conducted his assignment with the same perfection he brought to every task he undertook. He'd taken his revenge on Bucareli. Yet, I knew that in his heart he felt a deeper purpose. Cane had been king since the days of the Conquistadors. To Salvador, *la centrale* personified evil, holding his villagers in perpetual bondage, victims of the cruel twosome of debt and disease.

As the night brought darkness to the forest, Francesca fixed a bed for me on the utility room floor. Exhausted, I slept.

At first light, Francesca brought me a breakfast of coffee and bread and briefed me on the news of the battle as I ate. From what little I understood, I gathered that Marcos, Emilia, and the guerrillas had retreated only about half a mile into the forest before Marcos was able to mount a counterattack and drive Bucareli's troops out of Valencia and back across the *Ebro*.

The news was better than I'd hoped, but it only swelled the lump already present in my throat. Salvador could have jumped; we *both* would have escaped. Control of the upper road by Bucareli's forces probably ended only moments after the stunning flight of *Australorbis.*

With great fanfare, a crowd of village women walked with me down to the waiting school bus. With much excitement, they explained my plight to Felipe and to the kids who would be riding the bus with me.

In Comerio, after delivering the children to their school, Felipe left me locked in the bus for about half an hour, seated on the floor, concealed from prying eyes, my head resting against the rear bench seat. At one point I heard loud insistent voices outside the bus. Fearing we might be incorrectly parked, I expected any moment that an angry policeman might climb high enough to spot me there on the floor. I crawled between two seats on the left side of the aisle and lay there silently.

Felipe returned. At the very least, I expected him to report that I was wanted on charges of theft of government property, complicity in the destruction of the *centrale*, and engaging in covert activities in concert with the enemy. I was certain to be blindfolded and shot along with hundreds of other conspirators.

"What did you learn?" I asked.

"*Nada!*" he said. "Bucareli secret police look for many people. No look for *americano*."

"But would they know—the people you questioned?"

"They know, *señor*. Everybody know. You are hero in Comerio."

"So what do you recommend?"

"Maybe soldiers see you at Valencia. Bucareli find out soon. But okay now."

"My crew, my four workers joined the guerrillas."

"*Poco a poco* everybody join Marcos."

"I can't stay in Comerio. I'd soon be seen and caught."

"Take bus to Aguilas. You be okay."

"They'd arrest me at the ticket counter."

"Pay on bus. Is okay. You be okay."

As I stepped past him to leave he touched my arm. I turned. "*Buena suerte,*" he said.

I thanked him and left. I'm sure he breathed easier after I stepped down from the bus and slipped into the crowd at the bus terminal. No one accosted me as I waited to board the bus to Aguilas. Nor was anyone waiting to arrest me when I arrived at the city terminal. I walked the eight blocks to my hotel.

After a hot shower and a change of clothes, I decided to risk a quick trip to the office to collect some recent research data I had not had time to duplicate. My business suit covered my wounds, my face looked okay, and a bad cut on top of my head was well concealed by my hair.

Since the long Taviran arm of the law had not yet reached out to snare me, I thought it might be politically correct to check in with Gregorio. Such a move might help to defray suspicion in case any rumors might be floating around the Department of Health.

José Carrera raised his great bulk from the chair at his desk outside Palma's office, opened the office door, and announced my presence. To my surprise, I heard Bucareli's voice. Then Gregorio's as he told José to usher me in.

"Come and join us," Bucareli said. "We were just talking about you."

"Thank you," I said, adding, "Favorably, I hope?" I noticed that Luis and Charlie were in the room.

"Indeed yes," Bucareli said. "We are relieved to see you. We thought we had lost you for good. Luis said you told him you wanted to go the *centrale*, and we have worried that you might have been killed in the blast."

"You mean when *Centrale Allende* exploded?"

"Yes."

I glanced about the room. I caught Luis's eye. What else had he told them? If that's all he'd said, then I could improvise. But where did Luis imply that he last saw me? I felt it too risky to guess. Bucareli was fully capable of setting a trap for Luis and for me.

"Oh, I had a time, believe me!" I said. Then I pretended I was still eager to hear Luis's experience. "Luis," I asked, "where did you go after you left me?"

"I drove to the bridge, then straight home to Aguilas," he said. "Had trouble passing the tanks along the Ebro between Valencia and the bridge, but made it through okay."

He'd told me what I needed to know. I explained to the four of them that I was worried about Emilia, that I'd gone up into the woods to try to find her and my crew, and that all I managed to achieve was to almost get myself shot in the process of being captured.

"By the guerrillas?" Bucareli asked.

"Yes, three of them."

"And they let you go?" Bucareli asked with an expression of disbelief.

"This morning. Yes," I said. "After they counterattacked. I guess they felt quite magnanimous in view of their success."

It was tempting to describe for Bucareli the fabulous explosion of the *centrale*. What a masterful coup d'état to the day at Valencia. I could have described how the mushroom cloud blackened the sky two playing fields wide and all the way to Juncos to the east, how it incinerated four centuries of servitude and corruption while vaporizing half a ton of SCP to boot!

"Why did they let you go?" Bucareli asked.

"I don't know. They had my workers, Emilia, and me."

"Did they release Emilia?"

"No."

"Just you, alone?"

"Yes."

"Why? Who ordered your release?"

"A man who seemed to be in charge."

"Describe him." Bucareli seemed intent on debriefing me.

"A head shorter than me; late thirties; looked like all the others; no officer's insignia or anything like that."

"Did he say why he was releasing you?"

"Yes. He said I would be more use to him free than as a prisoner. I don't know what he meant by that, but I didn't hang around to ask."

"What did you want at *Centrale Allende*?" Bucareli asked.

"Absentee records," I said. "I wanted to try to determine how many work days are lost to schisto."

"The *centrale* would have had such records," Gregorio said, "but they've surely gone up in smoke. And here at the Department of Health we only have lab records of who at the plant has tested positive for schisto over the years."

"That alone wouldn't help much," I said.

The mention of the lab brought up again the capture of Emilia, and this tended to draw their attention from me. My mind raced over that issue, wondering what Luis would say about her. Would he admit to bringing her to Valencia? And why did she want to be there? I looked rather helplessly at Charlie. I could tell he was tense, but he picked up the baton anyway.

"Emilia phoned me last night," he said, almost casually. "Kept bugging me to drive her to Valencia." He looked at me. "Wanted to see how you carry out one of your follow-up surveys."

"Did you take her there?" Gregorio asked.

"I did," Luis said. "While Harvey and I fiddled around down by the *Ebro*, I noticed her talking to one of Harvey's crew. They were headed up along the *Segre*. That's the last I saw of her."

Bucareli turned to me. "Did it look to you as if they might mistreat her?"

"I don't know," I said. "I rather doubt it, actually. They seemed to be rather decent people and well disciplined."

"Perhaps we can negotiate her release," Bucareli said.

I'm sure Bucareli had many other questions. I'm sure he wasn't ready to let matters rest. Yet, somehow, he chose not to question me further. Instead, he ended the meeting abruptly—rather as though he had thought of something he needed to do.

"Well, gentlemen, I think we have about covered most of the points we need to discuss. Let me face this matter squarely and issue a proclamation that I'll expect you to honor. Since these hostilities may go on for a while longer, and I don't want more noncombatants injured or captured by these ruthless guerrillas, as of this minute I am putting the field program on hold. None of you is to attempt to conduct fieldwork of any sort whatsoever until you receive the okay from me personally.

"I'm freezing the program funds. No purchase orders are to leave Gregorio's desk, or even to be put on Gregorio's desk, for that matter. Actually, I expect it's likely that the government will decide to appropriate the project's funds. From the looks of things, we can expect to be running a deficit by the time we finish dealing with Marcos Díaz." He smiled and tried to create a little joke. "After all, we could reasonably define the search for *el señor* Díaz as a most urgent form of disease control."

None of us laughed. He rose from his chair. Then he turned briefly towards me. "I'm glad you are safe, Shoals." He frowned. "*Comprende?*"

I wondered what the *comprende* was supposed to imply. Coupled with the work stoppage, he could be hinting that my welcome on Tavira had run out.

Curiously, he stood around and seemed to want to sort of shoo us out of the room. My guess is that he didn't relish the thought of us sitting around disparaging the rout of his troops on their first skirmish with Marcos. And I'm sure he really did have urgent concerns: generals to demote to colonels, colonels to majors. *Etcetera*, as Luis might have added.

As we left the room, I asked Charlie quietly if we could talk over coffee at Rubie's.

"Better than that, lad," he said. "Come on home with me. We can't say all there is to say in Rubie's. Too many eyes and ears."

CHARLIE'S

As Charlie mixed a batch of martinis, he said, "I can't be certain, but if I were a gamblin' man, I'd wager Bucareli has a pretty good idea of my part in all of this. Of course, I'm not a Taviran citizen—although I've lived here so long I feel like one. But since I'm not, he can't get me for treason. He'll have to shoot me for something else.

"In any case, he will really need to have the goods on me. I've got clout enough with his supporters to survive most any public trial. Then there's the fact that I've got a buggerin' garbage can full of stuff on him."

"In that case, isn't it more likely, he'd have one of his henchmen kill you in the alley outside the warehouse some dark night?"

"I've been taking precautions. I try to be locked in at least by sunset."

"How did you get so involved in the first place with buying for Marcos?"

For a moment, I thought he wasn't going to tell me. Once he started, he touched on a number of questions that I needed to have answered.

"My wife Sally and I used to vacation here with our parents when we were kids. In fact, this is where we met. My dad was an importer. Built this building and the big warehouse east of us. I built the one on the right.

"Both Sally's parents and mine died in the forties and left us a passel of money. We got the idea of picking up just this end of my dad's business, and moving here from Atlanta to live the good life, as they say. Being importers was our way of boosting the economy and hopefully the standard of living on Tavira. We both loved it here and loved the people.

"Trouble was, we soon learned we were only satisfying the rich folk's craving for fancy stuff, we weren't doin' much for the ordinary folks or for the sugar cane workers out in the boondocks.

"Sally's hobbyhorse was to better the training of the destitute youth. She took what money she had left and started a technical school up near Comerio. Like to worked herself to death. In fact, in a way, maybe that's exactly what she did."

It was a bad joke. He looked at me apologetically. "No, actually, Sally couldn't stand the heat here in Aguilas. She chose Comerio to get up into a cooler climate. I love the heat. Hotter the better. But not Sally. Once, when she saw me working in the heat of the day, in hundred-degree weather, she said, 'You'll probably be the first human ever to escape from Hell.' We laughed a lot about that. She was a good soul. I miss her."

"When did she die?" I asked.

"Nineteen fifty-four."

"Is the school still there?"

"No. Began to go downhill soon as the Aggie Campus opened in Comerio."

"Where does Marcos enter the picture?"

"About 1951, Marcos opened a law office across the street from the school. He helped Sally with a bunch of legal stuff, and then he offered to teach business law. Sally got to know him an' Emilia both. We got interested in Marcos's efforts to oust Bucareli, but of course we never came out of the closet about that. When Bucareli fired Marcos's father and drove Marcos into the *Espoleta*, it just seemed natural that we help him all we could."

"Did Bucareli order the shooting of Hernando?" I asked.

"I *know* he did. I figure Bucareli judged Palma to be a serious contender in the election. You let a snake-oil salesman like Palma loose in those villages and he could sweep 'em off their feet. Come election time and he'd bus 'em to the polls in his damned spray trucks.

"The very day Pidal's legislation passed, I'll bet that's the day Bucareli decided to publicly discredit Palma. First the soldier platoons. Then if that didn't work—"

"Any proof?" I interrupted.

"Some. I figure he orders out the soldiers to make Palma look to be a wimp. Sends the signal that Palma's afraid of his own constituents . . . He tries that for a few months, but when it doesn't prove effective enough to suit him, he shoots some poor village kid . . . That works great. I'm surprised he didn't shoot a couple more."

"Who killed Palma?"

"You mean who ordered it, or who did the shooting?"

"The shooting."

"Those same two shooters plus four others, all from Bucareli's personal guard. I've got their names, but it would be my word against the six of them. Of course if Bucareli comes after me in court I maybe could do some trading . . . subpoena the shooters, plea-bargain—dredge up enough dirt to do some damage."

"So Bucareli saw a tempting way to take out Palma and blame Marcos?"

"Yep!"

"What *about* Marcos? Can he win?"

"Not only can he win, it would be awful hard for him to lose. I know what he's got. I should; I ordered every scrap of it. He's better armed than Russia. When the right opportunity comes along, he'll fight and he'll win."

"Where did he get the money for all that stuff?"

"That's the really bizarre part of the whole thing. Much of it comes from supporters in the States. So much of it, in fact, that every now and then Uncle Sam sends a few guys wearing tan topcoats to check it out. They generally hang around a while, do some snorkeling, scuba diving, eat a passel of seafood, then leave when they've lost their pocket money playing the slots.

"Mostly, it's Bucareli who asks Uncle Sam to send them. That's all Bucareli has to do is ask, and a couple of 'em show up on the afternoon flight. You have to understand that Uncle Sam has some mighty peculiar reasons for helping Bucareli stay in power. Some of it has to do with sugar, but the bulk of it has to do with Uncle Sam favoring the status quo over a newcomer with newfangled ideas. Better to support the devil himself than a dreamer with a carbine and a contemporary college education. You're seeing the same sort of thing with Batista's floundering regime in Cuba.

"In fact, our Uncle Sam has got some really weird hang-ups. You'll realize that as you get older. When it comes to recollecting what our own revolution was all about, you'll find our Uncle has got it tangled up with some of them senile dimensions." He grinned at me.

He knew that I knew that he was purposely embroidering his elocution with third-rate grammar. But it was fun to hear him do it. Of course, it may have been partly that third martini doing the talking.

"So Emilia is right, you're the wallet pincher," I said. "When she told me, I couldn't believe it. I couldn't see the connection."

"I feel like I have to keep score—narrow the risk, so to speak. I mean, suppose you'd been a federal agent on that plane from Puerto Rico. By now, you'd have been privy to all sorts of conversations between Emilia and Luis, even Marcos himself. You'd have nailed me to a cross in a heartbeat. Probably got a promotion for it, too.

"But to get back to your first question," Charlie added, "much of the money to supply Marcos is local. Surprisingly, not all the big, wealthy families on Tavira support Bucareli, not by a long shot. The lassitude of those others allowed him to win an election back in the thirties. Give a greedy man power and he'll use every tinklin' tuppence to entrench. That'll be his first priority, and that's exactly what Bucareli's done. Here it is twenty-five years later, and it's costing his disenchanted cronies twenty-five times as much to get him out of office as it did to get him in."

Charlie's upstairs living-quarters, in addition to bedroom and bath, had a large open sitting area that faced south. Huge French doors swung inward to reveal a white-enameled railing set into the doorjamb. Although this opening was not intended as a functional exit or entrance, there being no balcony, it served the marvelous purpose of letting a delicious breeze in from the sea. We sat in imported showroom chairs upholstered with a durable Scottish plaid, with our drinks in hand, and we watched schools of small fish in the harbor perform a ballet of synchronized leaps, each clearing the water by at least a foot in a perfect arc.

"Channel bass are after 'em," Charlie said. "There's always prey for the predators of this world. Finding a niche is not that hard."

The setting sun colored the bay a burning orange that gradually transformed to blood red. Potentially beautiful though it was, my mind's eye carried me back to Hernando and to that swath of crimson in the *Perico* as it flowed from the stone arch of the bridge to the boot of the forward rifleman. Again I saw their eyes meet; saw the nod that preceded the shots.

I reminded Charlie of our first encounter on the plane from Puerto Rico. *From what I gather*, he'd said, *you could need help—more of it than you can imagine!*

He tipped his martini glass ever so slightly in my direction. "I figured you looked a mite wet behind the ears for a federal agent. And if you were genuine—what you claimed to be—I had no doubt you'd eventually get yourself in trouble. As a matter of fact, you've got yourself in a heap a trouble."

"But if Bucareli suspects me, he didn't let on."

"Bucareli's biding his time. He has you in his sights but isn't sure which barrel to fire first. But the way you look today—what in Sam Hill cracked you on the top of your head—the way you've got yourself all buggered up, I'd say 'you been rode hard and put up wet.' What really happened back there in Valencia? I'm guessing you chose to accompany Salvador and *Australorbis's* on their final fateful journey, which explains why you didn't come home with Luis. But fill me in as to the details."

I choked up and couldn't muster anything to say except, "Salvador died."

Salvador's and my last moments in the truck were too private to want to share. And I'd already figured out why Charlie insisted on purchasing clumsy old *Australorbis*. There wasn't a shred of doubt in my mind that he and Marcos had outlined that chess move in detail months before the battle at Valencia. Only an army six-by would have enough room for a half-ton of SCP plus the bulky packing and padding for a dozen bottles of nitro, and also have strong enough springs and shocks for the punishing ride down that treacherous side road and over the edge of Allende Cliff.

Charlie must have noticed my tears. "Well, anyway," he said, "I'm betting you've discovered there's more to God's little paradise here than you bargained for."

He stopped talking long enough to reach for the decanter, and poured my glass needlessly full. The alcohol was beginning to dull the pain from a hundred cuts and bruises. Even so, I guessed where the conversation was headed.

"I've watched you kids come and go. Whether it's schisto, or malaria, or yellow fever, or yellow fever's little brother dengue, it's not so much what's in your bag of tricks that sets the stage for success or failure, it's more a case of how well you understand the politics of change."

His careless grammar had abruptly vanished. "I don't get you," I said. "What 'politics of change?'"

"Well, take Luis for example . . . Here's a family man in a culture that is just beginning to emerge from traditional roots. He sees the tender sprouts of change cropping up all around him in that scorched earth of the sugar cane fields. His kids dream of college in the States, but what does Luis do when he ought to be asserting his expertise even to the extent of backing you up in conferences with Palma? He tiptoes in, careful always not to antagonize *el jefe grande*, afraid to speak his mind.

"And out there in the field! He's thinking every day that he better be mighty careful not to accidentally wipe out the disease for good . . . What a pity if he inadvertently worked himself out of a job."

He scratched the back of his scalp and then pulled a pillow out from behind him in his overstuffed chair and tossed it across the room. "But take Palma, on the other hand—there's an entirely different genotype for you. He was raised on cabernet and linen napkins. He has a bigger appetite than Luis. He wastes no time finding a way to marinate his soul in pure, triple-distilled greed."

"And Bucareli?" I asked.

"Bucareli carries with him the seeds of his own destruction. There's a Marcos for each Bucareli that comes along. That may be the only positive thing a person can say in favor of the human race.

"Marcos will take care of Bucareli. It may take him a while, but Marcos will win if he doesn't get himself killed trying." He started then to talk about specific villagers in Juncos whom he knew, about Hernando's murder, and then back to Sally and her technical college where our discussion had begun.

As he talked, my mind reviewed the faces of the friends *I'd* made at Juncos and Valencia—especially the villagers on that enchanting night in Valencia when they saw living cercariae for the first time. As the one young mother said with such emotion, "Why no tell us something useful we can do? Why all time tell us what not to do?"

Given another set of circumstances at a different place and time, perhaps it might have fallen to me to be the one to tell her "something useful," to design a program of disease control that would conform to the realities of life as life was lived in those villages, one that would respect the villagers' intelligence and especially their rights.

At least Salvador knew that I had tried—Salvador, his hands gripping the oversized steering wheel of *Australorbis* with all the strength left in him, having to deal with his own private devil in a way thoroughly foreign to his gentle, incomparable skill.

I've never been sure just why he didn't jump. I felt so certain that he would. I suppose he stayed with *Australorbis* because, while descending that rocky, kidney jolting road, the old truck threatened to turn or flip or stall and thereby miss the mark.

I've been awakened in the night by his friendly rasping voice a thousand times in the many years since then. It was never intended as a question, but merely as a way to beg my attention when he would say, "*Doctor*, you know what happen?" And, inevitably, a wonderful optimism would come to dominate our hours together as he added, "Today we going to find a way."

# # #

Made in the USA
Monee, IL
05 November 2026

67383315R10109